6TH EDITION

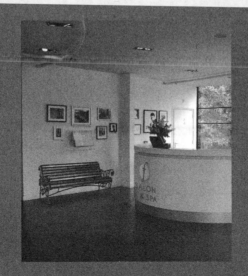

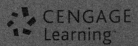
CENGAGE
Learning

EDWARD J. TEZAK
TERRY FOLAWN

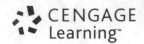

Successful Salon & Spa Management, Sixth Edition
Edward J. Tezak and Terry Folawn

President, Milady: Dawn Gerrain

Publisher: Erin O'Connor

Acquisitions Editor: Martine Edwards

Senior Product Manager: Phil Mandl

Editorial Assistant: Elizabeth Edwards

Director of Beauty Industry Relations:
Sandra Bruce

Senior Marketing Manager: Gerald McAvey

Production Director: Wendy Troeger

Senior Art Director: Joy Kocsis

Print Buyer: Charlene Taylor

Manufacturing Director: Martha Wallace

Content Project Management:
PreMediaGlobal

Cover Designer: Rokusek Design

Library of Congress Control Number: 2010939905

ISBN-13: 978-1-4354-8246-3

ISBN-10: 1-4354-8246-8

Milady
5 Maxwell Drive
Clifton Park, NY 12065-2919
USA

Cengage Learning is a leading provider of customized learning solutions with office locations around the globe, including Singapore, the United Kingdom, Australia, Mexico, Brazil, and Japan. Locate your local office at: **international.cengage.com/region**

Cengage Learning products are represented in Canada by Nelson Education, Ltd.

For your lifelong learning solutions, visit **milady.cengage.com**

Visit our corporate website at **cengage.com**

Printed in the United States of America
1 2 3 4 5 6 7 14 13 12 11 10

Contents

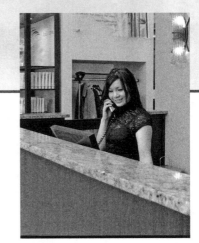

■ Chapter 1

■ Chapter 2

Chapter 13

Preface

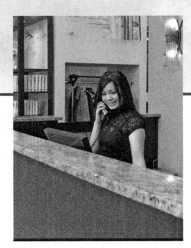

When I was asked to rewrite the sixth edition of *Successful Salon and Spa Management*, I was excited to have the privilege to enhance and update the originally published text. I really enjoyed the step-by-step manner in which it had been written and had to ask myself if I truly felt I could not only update the information but add valuable content as well. My many years of experience in the salon and spa industry have given me a broad perspective of what it really takes to simplify the process of opening and running a business. I have written the sixth edition with the intent of taking the mystery out of opening a salon or spa business. Anyone—from the wide-eyed new entrepreneur to the seasoned business owner—will find tools and systems that are easy to follow and implement.

The truth in today's ever-changing world is that the vast majority of businesses will fail within two years of opening their doors. Most of the survivors, despite their potential, will soon follow, either suffering from a chronically low profit margin (a slow and agonizing death) or cleverly juggling only to close their doors a few years later. It is an unfortunate truth that 90 percent of small businesses in the United States close within the first five years.

That being said, the one essential difference between the businesses that fall into this gloomy statistic and a business that survives and prospers is...

◖ PLANNING!

As the old saying goes, "**He who fails to plan, plans to fail!**"

The beauty industry is often credited with being one of the most rapidly growing industries today. In the pages ahead, you will find a comprehensive, systematic guide to opening and running a successful salon and spa. The use of this book should simplify the process of opening a new business or getting your existing business on track. We have all said, at one time or another, "If I only knew then what I know now."

This book chronicles the foundations of opening a salon and spa, detailing how to choose the type of salon and spa you want, the location, how to finance your new business, and every decision in between. It seems that every hairstylist or beauty technician who graduates from cosmetology school dreams of opening his or her own salon and spa. Students today are exposed to a much more sophisticated education than was available even ten years ago. Graduates believe they are prepared for anything after completing the required hours and receiving a license. Many are creative and talented individuals, but it takes more than a great technician to run a salon and spa business successfully. There are many aspects of opening a salon and spa, and you will find that this book will serve as a guide to support you with those details.

There are many serious questions you need to ask yourself before beginning the journey of becoming a small business owner. What type of salon and spa business do you want? What are the differences between a salon and a spa? Are you prepared for a large investment of time and money? What are your short- and long-term goals, both personally and professionally?

WHAT'S NEW IN THIS EDITION

Beginning with financing the project, Chapters 1–2 clearly defines the different financial options. Your salon and spa business will require financing to grow. Often, lenders are very aware that these businesses can and will struggle with the cost of varying receivables and high overhead. The success of your salon and spa is based on a local "loyal" following, and until your business has time to establish its "regulars," revenue can be very unstable, making it difficult to repay your fixed loan. The banks are well aware of this; being prepared is the answer.

Next you'll need to know how to actually operate your salon and spa for a profit once you have it up and running (Chapters 3–5). These chapters include great basic information on operating cost, permits, insurances, and rental/lease agreements, all of which are the foundations of operating at a margin that will allow you to make a profit and keep your doors open for years to come. (We can look at businesses in any field and find ones that are thriving and ones that are failing. The key is planning and understanding your business.)

We also cover trial-and-error decoration and placement questions in Chapters 6–7. Decorating may seem like the easy part of the process; however, it can be very time-consuming and a financial money pit if done without detailed planning.

At this point in the book, you should have the foundation of a tangible business—and the foundation is what will keep you strong in the long run. But there is more to learn.

Lastly, you will need staff and clients, as what good is a business if you don't have a great staff to run it or clients to patronize it? This is where Chapters 8–13, which talk about management tools, salon and spa record-keeping, marketing, product selection, and creating working relationships with cosmetology schools, come in handy—each will help you to attract the type of staff as well as the clients you desire for your business.

SUPPLEMENTS

The *Workbook to Accompany Successful Salon and Spa Management*, sixth edition, contains many useful guided questions based on specific areas of study discussed in this text. Because it was designed to coordinate with the text, you will be able to turn to the exact section in both in order to complete your work.

I also encourage you to always search out new tools and books to help you in your business. Milady has a plethora of resources for the salon or spa manager, including financial tools, management training, one-on-one coaching, and so much more. To find out the latest information, visit http://milady.cengage.com.

As you step forward into your business journey, it is my hope that you will view this book as a set of business guidelines. It is important that you become thoroughly informed about all aspects of the salon and spa business. If you are interested in either beginning or improving your business skills, this step-by-step guide will help place you in a prime position to achieve business success.

Stay informed, keep a sense of humor, and keep your chin up!

About the Authors

Edward J. Tezak has spent over 50 years as a professional in the barber/ beauty industry. His career started as a barber and later as a barbershop owner. Advanced studies in the industry found Mr. Tezak as a hairstylist, salon manager of a major chain, salon owner, and later an instructor of cosmetology in both private and public educational institutions. Mr. Tezak holds a B.Ed., M.Ed in education along with certifications in special needs students, curriculum development, and teacher mentoring. Mr. Tezak has taught nationally and internationally, and written several articles for professional journals both in cosmetology/barbering and education. He has served on national boards for cosmetology and barbering, evaluation, and licensure. More recently he has served as an examiner for both cosmetology and barbering in the state of Colorado for licensing purposes.

Successful Salon and Spa Management is used throughout the United States as a management textbook and has been translated into five languages. Presently the textbook is used in several countries throughout the world.

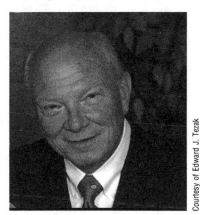

Edward J. Tezak

Courtesy of Edward J. Tezak

Terry Folawn has over 30 years of experience in the beauty industry as a stylist, trainer, manager, and business owner.

She is the owner of The Spa @ Folawn's in San Antonio, Texas, a premier salon and spa for over 17 years.

One of Terry's most cherished accomplishments is a charity event she and her daughter started in 2004 and run to support the fight against child abuse, named My Princess and Me.

Terry truly believes that continuing education, professionalism, and an unwavering belief in the human sprit will remain the determining factors to make us successful.

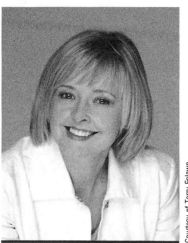

Terry Folawn

Courtesy of Terry Folawn.

Reviewers

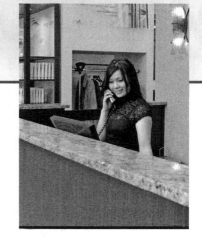

I would like to thank the following individuals in particular who reviewed the sixth edition and offered insightful comments and suggestions during its writing. Reviewing can be a time-consuming task, but it is critical to the success of the book. I am deeply grateful to each of you for your time and your comments.

Sheryl Baba
Solstice Day Spa
Cape Cod, MA

Sharon Bethel
Eastland Career Center
Groveport, OH

Jessica Cummings
Face Forward Inc.
Peabody, MA

Corrinne Denise Edwards
Temple Hills, MD

Caryl Ann Johnson
International Academy
of Hair Design
Scottsdale, AZ

Fredrick J. Laurino
House of Heavilin of Kansas,
Inc., Wichita, KS

Suzanne Mathis McQueen
The Phoenix,
an Aveda Concept

Salon & Spa
Ashland, OR

Stella M. Niffenegger
The Hornsby Group
Cincinnati, OH

Kathy Phelps
Norman, OK

Ada Polla
Alchimie Forever
Washington DC

Linda Riley, Miami
Correctional Facility
Barber School,
Walton, IN

Nancy Schmidt
Capital Region Career and
Tech School,
Pattersonville, NY

Vincenza Tamaro
Ohio Academy,
Twinsburg, OH

Melanie Thompson
Myrtle Beach, SC

Nadine Toriello
All About You
Day Spa, Keys To Esthetics
and Monroe County Adult
Education Esthetics Licensing
Program
Key West, FL

Regena (Gena) Walters
Ehove Career Center
Milan, OH

Kenneth Young
Hotheads Hair Design
Oklahoma City, OK

Acknowledgments

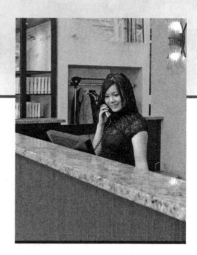

The Successful Salon Managements series was designed to help guide entrepreneurs into successful business ownership. My many years of experience in creating and owning businesses have brought me a great understanding of the importance of planning first and jumping second.

I'd like to thank Edward J. Tezak for writing the foundations of *Successful Salon and Spa Management* and allowing me an opportunity to update the information, creating relevance for today's entrepreneurs.

Additional thanks goes to those who spent numerous hours contributing to the series.

Photography:
- Dino Petrocelli

Edits:
- Abigail Perrine | Development Manager

Production:
- Arul Joseph Raj | Project Manager

And a final thanks, to the ones without whom my life would have no meaning.

I'd like to acknowledge my husband, Ken, who has been an incredible strong shoulder to cry on and a best friend to laugh with. I'm not sure what I would do without your undying support.

To my children, Alexx and Hailee, you are the joy of my life. Your laughter makes everything else seem less significant.

I am grateful to Elizabeth and Laura, for your endless hours of proofreading.

Salon and Spa Types and Their Locations

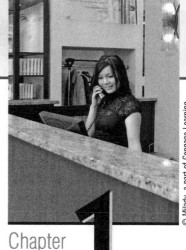

© Milady, a part of Cengage Learning.
Photography by Dino Petrocelli

Chapter **1**

INTRODUCTION

Ownership of a business and the operation of that business require a different set of skills from those associated with a given trade or profession. The first step in successfully entering the business side of the beauty industry requires a series of well-thought-out decisions. The first five chapters of this text are designed to give the first-time **entrepreneur** and the seasoned owner a step-by-step approach to setting up the business.

At one time, beauty salons and barber shops were simple, small operations, from one to four people. The business side was often operated solely by the owner, who hired professional, fully licensed trade employees. Women traditionally went to the beauty salon and men to the barber shop. The states licensed these technicians in all areas particular to their profession. Today, a series of **sublicenses** are issued by most states. Some alternative or special licenses, such as massage therapy, may or may not be honored by other licensing entities throughout the country. Each of the states has different requirements concerning the practice of the cosmetology industry and the operation of establishments who render service to the public.

The first step is to read and follow the licenses required for business ownership. In most cases, those regulations are found in the department of regulatory agencies at the state capital. The "laws" governing the beauty industry will state what establishments can conduct what activities within a given region, by whom, and under what conditions. An example follows from the Barber & Cosmetology Act in 2005 of the state of Colorado:

> "**Place of business**" means a fixed establishment, temporary location, or place, including any mobile barber or beauty salons, in which one or more

entrepreneur

A person who has possession of a new enterprise, venture, or idea and assumes significant accountability for the inherent risks and the outcome.

sublicense

A license giving rights to occupy a rented space to a person or company that is not the primary holder of such location.

place of business

A fixed establishment, temporary location, or place, including any mobile barber or beauty salon, in which one or more persons practice as barbers, hairstylists, cosmetologists, manicurists, or estheticians.

temporary location
A location that is not permanent for your business. A term that denotes a finite period of time, with a defined beginning and an end.

freestanding salon and spa
A salon and spa whose structure is not attached to another structure.

persons engage in the practice of barbering, hair styling, cosmetology, or practice as a manicurist or esthetician. The term "**temporary location**" includes a motor home as defined in Section 41-2-102 (57) CSR.

Once you have a firm grasp of the law, you need to determine exactly what services your establishment will offer (including start-up services and future services as the salon and spa changes year to year). Do you need to offer all salon services in your establishment, or can the salon and spa offer only a few services? (Example: a "haircut salon" that offers haircutting only). Can a salon offer a barber service "shaving" under a beauty salon license, or does another license need to be acquired even if the service is rendered by a licensed barber within the state and in the licensed salon and spa?

Permanent makeup, laser hair removal, tattooing, piercing, hair extensions, chemical facial peels, braiding, and removal of calluses, corns, and ingrown nails have generated much discussion at the regulatory-agency level over the last few years. The only true, hard fact is that each state regulates the industry in the state, and all state regulations are different.

The second step is to write all salon and spa services you wish to offer in the establishment. The list should not list the services the owner wants to perform, but those services that should be offered to the public because of location and economic, ethnic, and age dynamics. For example: You would not want to specialize in children's haircuts if the salon and spa is in a retirement home.

Next, see what licenses are needed to be able to carry out these services and how the establishment should be licensed. Note that sales of items and products such as shampoo, hair spray, facial cream, nail polish, brushes, combs, and blow dryers can make up from 20 percent to 50 percent of the overall income of a salon and spa. Most states require a sales tax license for these items. A sales tax license can usually be obtained from the Department of Revenue in the state where the salon and spa is located.

WHAT TYPE OF SALON AND SPA DO YOU WANT?

In general, five types of locations for salons and spas are used:

1. Hotel salons and spas
2. Department store/fitness center salons and spas
3. Mall/Shopping center salons and spas
4. **Freestanding salons and spas**
5. Medical spas

Hotel Salons and Spas

Today, hotels/resorts are designed to house major conventions and seminars. They may or may not be near a major retail establishment such as a downtown area. Those stand-alone resorts/hotels may be several miles from a retail outlet. The hotel offsets this lack of shopping activity by expansion of the salon and spa into a day spa. The services range from hair services to full-body massage, makeup, hair removal, body wraps, Botox injections, manicure, acrylic nails, pedicures, false eyelashes, permanent makeup, and a host of other services. While these services are done in a confined area, not all services are controlled by the cosmetology/barber board; some are controlled by the medical board. Should you wish to become an owner, partner, or associate in one of these establishments, be sure you conform to all laws governing such services. Contracts or lease agreements for hotel/spa space may contain certain unusual clauses, some of which are stated here:

1. Restrictions may be placed on where signs may be placed and what size and type of sign you may use.
2. Cleaning and maintenance work may be provided by the hotel, but charged back to the owner in addition to rent. In cases in which the establishment decides which cleaning firm does the maintenance work, be sure you know who has the right of supervision and control. There have been cases where the salon and spa owner had no control over when the cleaning was to be done, how thorough it was, or how long the cleaning staff would work.
3. A charge system is sometimes in effect that allows hotel guests to charge beauty/spa services to their overall hotel tab. In such cases, the hotel will make adjustments to the salon and spa in the form of cash refunds or rent credit to the salon and spa.
4. In some cases, hours during which the establishment is open or closed are regulated by the hotel contract.
5. Decorating can be a problem if there is a clause in the agreement giving the hotel the right to veto a salon and spa decorating plan if the hotel feels it will not go well with the other furnishings and decorations found in the hotel.
6. Since the new spa offers services that are not controlled by the cosmetic industry, such as permanent cosmetics, Botox, and so forth, a subcontractor clause should be written. This gives the salon and spa the right to secure the noncosmetic services, on an individual-contractor basis, free of control from the hotel management.
7. As with all contracts in which space is leased, you should have in writing how disputes regarding customer service are charged and

settled. The hotel is usually far more flexible in the return-of-product area (even if it has been opened and used) than the salon and spa. In some cases, the manager discounts a salon and spa service that the patron thinks is too expensive. Be extremely careful of this clause. You may wish to have your attorney carefully look over this section of your lease.

Department Store/Fitness Center Salons and Spas

While department stores have expanded the cosmetic, false-hair goods, and jewelry areas, the actual labor-intensive area of the salon and spa has become less popular in the past few years; however, they are still a viable option. Fitness centers are similar in concept. The salon and spa is located within the business and relies on the department store/fitness center for clients, marketing, and so forth.

The department store salon and spa and fitness center usually operates in a leased-space area. Major department stores and fitness centers usually contract with a nationwide chain of salons and spas, and their operations can vary from a small salon and spa to a multiunit salon and spa of 30 to 60 technicians. The chain makes its profit by mass purchasing and central supply depots. When a salon and spa needs a product, the home office is contacted, and the supplies are delivered. The supplies for this type of operation are usually ordered once a month, and each salon is well-supplied with products. The waste in so ordering is offset by mass purchasing and special sales run at slow periods of the year to reduce over-stocking merchandise, thereby disposing of products that are outdated.

All department store and fitness center salons and spas have certain things in common; for instance, the store usually supplies an accounting system and audit facility. The space in the store is usually rented or leased on a long-term contract, with a base rent, and a percentage of sales after a certain gross figure are reached. An additional fee is charged for the cost of accounting and maintenance.

Some major factors to consider before owning or managing a department store or fitness center salon and spa are:

1. The image and clientele of the department store must be absolutely compatible with the client you want for the salon and spa. The department store will draw the clients for you; it does not work the other way around.
2. You need to know how much marketing the store will be doing during the year. A store with a lot of traffic and high gross sales figures will deliver more prospective customers to your salon and spa than a store that is keeping just ahead of **bankruptcy**.

bankruptcy
When an individual or company has been declared, by law, to be unable to pay its debts to creditors or individuals.

3. Who has the final word on complaints and adjustments that are part of day-to-day business? The store manager is much more likely than the salon and spa manager to refund a customer the money paid for work received, even if the work is of good quality. The store manager's reasoning may take into consideration the fact that while the store suffers the loss of the percentage of a salon and spa service, the **customer's goodwill** may benefit the store in the long run. You may want to have more control over these situations, so definite rules should be set up for this in your contract.

4. In a department store salon and spa, who will do the hair of the fashion models hired for style shows? When should notice be given? What will the charge or credit for this service be? Answers should be in your contract. In dealing with models, the hairstyle should be approved by the salon and spa's style director with the cooperation of the fashion show coordinator.

5. As with all business negotiations, such things as employee benefits, parking permits for employees, parking permits for customers, credit cards, accounting procedures, decoration coordination, marketing, and actual production time (store hours) should be clearly stated and fully understood by the manager and the salon and spa manager and/or owner.

customer's goodwill
The value of intangible assets such as a strong brand name, good customer relations, and good employee relations.

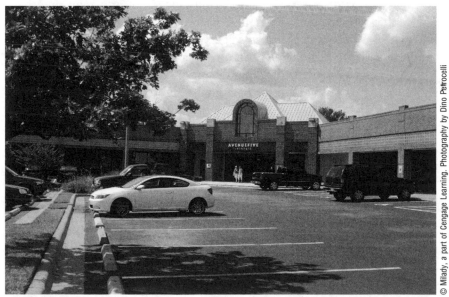

Shopping Center Location.

© Milady, a part of Cengage Learning. Photography by Dino Petrocelli

employee discount
Often used as incentive to work for a company, a discount on services or a percentage off products.

Employees of department store and fitness center salons and spas enjoy some important benefits that other salons and spas do not offer: the use of a store lunchroom or cafeteria, **employee discounts**, paid vacation, sick pay (sometimes), group insurance, and, in some cases, a profit-sharing program involving all store employees. The salon and spa often has the advantage of national and local store-paid marketing of beauty products and salon and spa services. As with all services and benefits offered to the employee, the salon and spa must in some way carry its own share of the financial responsibility.

Mall/Shopping Center Salons and Spas

Within a mall, a salon and spa can rely on convenience for the consumers; often malls are designed around a central atrium; they have numerous other businesses for your customer convenience and entertainment, such as movie theaters, restaurants, fast-food outlets, and public areas.

Within a shopping center, a salon and spa can rely on the convenience of a collection of independent retail stores and services much like the mall. Normally they are placed in one long strip center with a vast sea of parking lots. Giving the consumer the ability to go directly into your businesses without having to walk into a mall setting.

The size of this type of salons and spas will vary; it usually has from two to eight technicians. But, depending on the size of the center, it may contain more.

The rent is determined by a leasing agreement and may involve a flat rent plus a percentage figure after a certain level of gross sales is reached. Percentage of gross sales varies according to the length of time the shopping center has been in operation but usually is between 8 and 15 percent. (This is more commonly found in a mall than a shopping center.) The base (or flat) rent is figured on a square-foot-per-year basis. For example, a salon and spa 30 feet by 70 feet has 2,100 square feet. At $10 per square foot, the annual base rent is $21,000 a year, or $1,750 a month. Keep in mind that the dollar amount per square foot will vary greatly depending on city and location.

Mall/Shopping centers may operate on a multiyear lease with a "cost-of-operation" clause. This allows the rent to increase or decrease as the economy of the community changes due to inflation or depression. This enables the landlord to raise or lower the rent and the price of certain services without suffering any major loss of profit from investment.

Rent can vary greatly depending on the location, the type of mall, and the state of the economy, and you may be charged a percentage of your rent or space cost for mall upkeep, especially in an enclosed mall. Before deciding on a mall location, remember that all malls are not created equal. Like department stores, malls may have an orientation toward a particular type of shopper, for example, price-conscious as opposed to quality-conscious, or young and trendy as opposed to older and more classically conservative. And, while a strip mall does not give you the guaranteed traffic found in an enclosed mall, being stuck at the end of a little-traveled extension in an enclosed mall would put you out of the mainstream and would definitely affect your walk-in business.

The best way to handle negotiations for rent and other costs in a mall/shopping center is to know the location very well: **demographics**, traffic patterns, seasonal considerations, and so forth. Then, hire an attorney or business consultant familiar with such negotiations to help you through the process. This will speed up the process and give you the assurance of getting the best deal possible.

In most shopping centers and strip malls, an association of all shop owners is usually formed. The association dues are one major difference between a **privately owned salon and spa** and a shopping center salon and spa. Each usually owns his or her own business and has his or her own problems. The association helps to solve the common problems of doing business, such as snow removal, liability insurance, parking lot lighting, trash collection, and sometimes, window washing, known as *common area maintenance*. The association affords the individual shop-keeper a cooperative marketing program in which, for example, the entire center may run a full-page ad as a sales promotion three or four times a year. Christmas decoration for the center can be coordinated by this association, and mutual landlord problems can be effectively handled.

When a shopping center opens, the landlord usually provides space for a salon and spa. This space is contracted for by square footage. It should be large enough for expansion but small enough to operate profitably. A newly built center versus a well-established center will provide different challenges. A new center, commonly called a "white box," will have the following:

1. A floor (usually made of cement suitable for covering with stain, tile, carpet, or wood)
2. Four walls (usually prepared for painting); the support construction tolerance and blueprint of your equipment installation should be analyzed prior to lease signing
3. A ceiling (this is usually left rough but suitable to house a drop-tile ceiling)
4. Some type of toilet facility (usually a toilet and sink left exposed)
5. Heating or air-conditioning capabilities (no ductwork)
6. Electrical connections to the area (no wiring work)
7. A display window and a front and back door for customer service

demographics
The profiles of characteristics of a population used in government, marketing, or opinion research.

privately owned salon and spa
A business arrangement in which the owner has total and unlimited personal liability for profit or debts incurred by the business.

Note: All of the preceding provisions are regulated by the state and the county in which you live. Check your local laws, rules, and regulations.

A previously owned salon and spa may be a more cost-effective alternative because much of the work may have already been done for you, but keep in mind that there are pros and cons, and that it is important to know how to work with what you have got. In most cases, landlords will provide a small building allowance for additional improvements.

Freestanding Salons and Spas

In the freestanding salon and spa, the corporation or partnership owns the property. With this arrangement:

1. The salon and spa becomes more valuable day by day as the rent, which would otherwise be paid out, is used to pay for the purchase of the land and the building. The salon and spa is worth the price of the equipment, the price of supplies on hand, investment for utilities (electrical wiring, plumbing, etc.), and the value of the land and building less the amount of any mortgage involved.
2. The landlord–salon and spa owner arrangement is also quite common. In this case, the property is owned and maintained by a person who is also the owner and technician of the salon and spa. This landlord–salon and spa owner owns the land and building, a part of which he or she leases for a salon and spa. He then charges rent to the salon and spa. The value of the salon and spa in this case reflects only the cost of the actual business and not the cost of the structure that houses it.
3. If the owner of the salon and spa and property lives in the residence, part of which is used for the salon and spa, salon and spa expenses are tax-deductible in proportion to the percentage of space occupied by the salon and spa.

Note: Due to our present tax structure, it is wise to consult a good accountant or tax official to find out the best way to set up your accounts in order to take fullest advantage of allowable tax deductions.

The home salon and spa while less common today, I do feel is worth mentioning. This type of location is commonly not larger than four to five stations. The cost of starting such an establishment is quite low, and supplies can be purchased as they are needed. The salon and spa owner/manager is usually the "jack-of-all-trades": the front desk associate, the technician, the repairman, the bookkeeper, the cleaning crew, the manicurist, the public-relations person, and the supply room clerk. As a result, the percentage of profit shown by a small operation is the highest in our industry, at the cost of a heavier workload and a reduced amount of the owner/manager's free time.

Medical Spas

The "medical spa" began to be introduced in the United States in 1997 by a group of innovative doctors. Its concept combines Western and holistic medicine combined with spa services to create a relaxing luxurious atmosphere. You must have a physician's license to open a medical spa; however, you may choose to join forces with a physician in order to offer medical services. Some of these services may include: Botox, laser hair removal, chemical peels, Restylane, and dermatological services.

 ## WHO OWNS THE SALON AND SPA?

Several ownership arrangements have developed in the past several years. They range from sole proprietorships to a corporation type of arrangement.

Sole Proprietorships

The vast majority of small businesses start out as **sole proprietorships**. These firms are owned by one person, usually the individual who has day-to-day responsibility for running the business. Sole proprietors own all the assets of the business and the profits generated by it. They also assume complete responsibility for any of its liabilities or debts. In the eyes of the law and the public, you and the business are one and the same.

sole proprietorship
A business arrangement in which a single individual owns all the assets of the business, including the profits generated by it, and assumes all responsibilities for any of the liabilities or debts.

Advantages

- The sole proprietorship is the easiest and least expensive form of ownership to organize.
- Sole proprietors are in complete control, and within the parameters of the law, may make decisions as they see fit.
- Sole proprietors receive all income generated by the business, to keep or reinvest at their discretion.
- Profits from the business flow directly to the owner's personal tax return.
- The business is easy to dissolve, if desired.

Disadvantages

- Sole proprietors have unlimited liability and are legally responsible for all debts against the business. Their business and personal assets are at risk.

- May be at a disadvantage in raising funds, and are often limited to using funds from personal savings or consumer loans.
- Some employee benefits such as owner's medical insurance premiums are not directly deductible from business income; they are only partially deductible as an adjustment to income.

Partnerships

partnership

A form of business in which two or more people operate for the common goal of making profit. Each partner has unlimited liability for all debts and profits of the business.

In a **partnership**, two or more people share ownership of a single business. Like proprietorships, the law does not distinguish between the business and its owners. The partners should have a legal agreement that sets forth how decisions will be made, how profits will be shared, how disputes will be resolved, how future partners will be admitted to the partnership, how partners can be bought out, and what steps will be taken to dissolve the partnership when needed. Yes, it is hard to think about a breakup when the business is just getting started, but many partnerships split up at times of crisis, and unless there is a defined process, there will be even greater problems. They also must decide up front how much time and capital each will contribute, and so forth.

Advantages

- Partnerships are relatively easy to establish; however, time should be invested in developing the partnership agreement.
- With more than one owner, the ability to raise funds may be increased.
- Prospective employees may be attracted to the business if given the incentive to become a partner.
- The business usually will benefit from partners who have complementary skills.

Disadvantages

- Partners are jointly and individually liable for the actions of the other partner(s).
- Profits must be shared with others.
- Since decisions are shared, disagreements can occur.
- The partnership may have a limited life; it may end upon the withdrawal or death of a partner.

Types of Partnerships to Consider

1. General Partnership   Partners divide responsibility for management and liability, as well as the shares of profit or loss, according to their internal agreement. Equal shares are assumed unless there is a written agreement that states differently.

2. Limited Partnership and Partnership with Limited Liability   *Limited* means that most of the partners have limited liability (to the extent of their investment) as well as limited input regarding management decisions, which generally encourages investors for short-term projects or for investing in capital assets. This form of ownership is not often used for operating retail or service businesses. Forming a limited partnership is more complex and formal than forming a **general partnership**.

3. Joint Venture   Is like a general partnership, but is clearly for a limited period of time or a single project. If the partners in a **joint venture** repeat the activity, they will be recognized as an ongoing partnership and will have to file as such, as well as distribute accumulated partnership assets upon dissolution of the entity.

Corporations

A **corporation** chartered by the state in which it is headquartered is considered by law to be a unique entity, separate and apart from those who own it. A corporation can be taxed, it can be sued, and it can enter into contractual agreements. The owners of a corporation are its shareholders. The shareholders elect a board of directors to oversee the major policies and decisions. The corporation has a life of its own and does not dissolve when ownership changes.

Advantages

- Shareholders have limited liability for the corporation's debts or judgments against the corporations.
- Generally, shareholders can only be held accountable for their investment in stock of the company. (Note, however, that officers can be held personally liable for their actions, such as the failure to withhold and pay employment taxes.)
- Corporations can raise additional funds through the sale of stock.
- A corporation may deduct the cost of benefits it provides to officers and employees.
- S corporation status can be elected if certain requirements are met. This election enables the company to be taxed similar to a partnership.

Disadvantages

- The process of incorporation requires more time and money than other forms of organization.

general partnership

A business arrangement in which partners divide responsibility for management and liability, as well as the shares of profit or loss, according to their internal agreement. Equal shares are assumed unless there is a written agreement that states differently.

joint venture

A legal entity formed between two or more parties to undertake an economic activity together, like a general partnership but clearly for a limited period of time or a single project.

corporation

An institution that is granted a charter recognizing it as a separate legal entity having its own privileges, and liabilities distinct from those of its members.

- Corporations are monitored by federal, state, and some local agencies, and as a result may have more paperwork to comply with regulations.
- *Incorporating* may result in higher overall taxes. Dividends paid to shareholders are not deductible from business income; thus, they can be taxed twice.

Subchapter S Corporations

An election as an "**S corporation**" is a tax election only; this election enables the shareholder to treat the earnings and profits as distributions and have them pass through directly to his or her personal tax return. The catch here is that if the shareholder is working for the company and there is a profit, the shareholder must pay himself or herself wages, and these must meet the standards for "reasonable compensation." This can vary by geographical region as well as occupation, but the basic rule is to pay yourself what you would have to pay someone to do your job, as long as there is enough profit. If you do not do this, the Internal Revenue Service (IRS) can reclassify all earnings and profit as wages, and you will be liable for all payroll taxes on the total amount.

Limited Liability Company (LLC)

The **LLC** is a relatively new type of hybrid business structure that is now permissible in most states. It is designed to provide the limited-liability features of a corporation and the tax efficiencies and operational flexibility of a partnership. Formation is more complex and formal than that of a general partnership. The owners are members, and the duration of the LLC is usually determined when the organization papers are filed. The time limit can be continued at the time of expiration, if desired, by a vote of the members. LLCs must not have more than two of the four characteristics that define corporations: limited liability to the extent of assets, continuity of life, centralization of management, and free transferability of ownership interests.

Franchised Salons and Spas

Franchised salons and spas have expanded significantly over the last 15 years, such as Fantastic Sam's, SuperCuts, and Visible Changes. Like food franchise operations (such as McDonald's), these have been very successful because of their marketing and organizational strengths.

Although most of these franchises are locally owned by individuals, some are in fact owned by the franchise company. Regardless, a franchise offers standardization. Management operations and services are all done

S corporation

For U.S. federal income-tax purposes, a corporation that makes a valid election to be taxed under Subchapter S of Chapter 1 of the Internal Revenue Code. In general, S corporations do not pay any federal income taxes. Instead, the corporation's income or losses are divided among and passed through to its shareholders.

limited liability company (LLC)

A business arrangement that provides the limited-liability features of a corporation and the tax efficiencies and operational flexibility of a partnership.

under strict guidelines to ensure a certain level of quality. D cor is standard, as are the products sold and even the design of the salon and spa.

Although such an operation would seem stifling to some people, it has certain advantages.

Advantages

- Strong consumer marketing
- Group purchasing power
- Uniform bookkeeping systems
- Centralized training
- Zones guarantee noncompetition from other salons and spas in the same franchise
- Exclusivity of product line
- Help with interior design
- Legal and business assistance programs at a reduced cost
- Group insurance rates for malpractice and liability
- In some cases, group health insurance for employees

Disadvantages

- You may find that your costs are higher than you originally expect. Not only will you have the initial costs of purchasing the franchise, you maybe required to pay continuing management service fees, as along with having to buy products directly from the franchisor.
- A franchise agreement commonly includes several restrictions on how you run the business. You may find yourself not being able to make the changes you deem better suited for your local market.
- The franchisor might go out of business.
- Other franchisees could give the brand a less then desirable reputation. The consumer sees you as one and the same.
- You may find it difficult to sell your franchise; Remember you bought into a brand, so all potential buyers would first have to be approved by the franchisor.
- All profits are shared with the franchisor
- You may find that your costs are higher than you expect. Not only will you have the costs of buying the franchise, you may pay continuing management service fees, and you may have to agree to buy products from the franchisor.
- The franchise agreement usually includes certain restrictions on how you run the business. You might not be able to make changes you deem better suited for your local market.

- The franchisor might go out of business.
- Other franchisees could give the brand a bad reputation. The consumer sees you as one and the same.
- You may find it difficult to sell your franchise; all potential buyers would first have to be approved by the franchisor.
- All profits are shared with the franchisor.

Employee-Owned Corporations

Employee stock-ownership plans offer some unique advantages. In this type of arrangement, the employees own stock in the company, which they purchase when the company is formed or which they earn as part of their compensation over the years.

A cooperative venture works best when the members know how to work together, of course, and when they realize that compromise is essential. Although not very common, employee ownership is a viable alternative, but only if the personalities involved are compatible. Even with stock being evenly distributed, however, one or two people usually emerge as leaders. In reality, even the most agreeable people will have difficulty running a successful salon and spa as a group without the strong guidance of a leader to give the business direction and consistency.

Advantages
- Motivate employees to become more productive
- Align employees' interests with those of shareholders
- Recruit or retain key employees
- Compensate for lower salaries and relieve pressure on cash flow
- Remunerate employees in a tax-efficient way
- Increase loyalty and reduce staff turnover
- Raise working capital
- Realize owners' investment

Disadvantages
- The effect on morale and retention if the share price falls—particularly for share option schemes
- Administration costs—short-term costs of drawing up and getting a scheme approved, plus long-term costs of managing the scheme and keeping records
- Dilution of share ownership—as more shares are issued, each share you own becomes a smaller percentage of the company; you could lose control of the business

- Risks of arousing among employees unrealistic expectations of the financial rewards
- If employees eventually wish to sell their shares in an unlisted company (one without shares on a public stock exchange), having to run an internal market for the shares, perhaps through setting up an employee benefit trust

Leased Space and Booth Rental

The latest ownership models are the leased-space salon and spa cooperative. In this model, the owner contracts for a given area of space. The owner may own the building or lease space from a real estate entity, such as a shopping center or separate building in a stand-alone arrangement. The owner subdivides the space into several areas. In its original form the area is divided into several rooms or studios, much like a doctor's office. Each room is rented to a practitioner for a service. When you follow the booth-rental business model, you are in effect just a landlord.

Advantages

- You do not pay workers' compensation or federal and state employment taxes.
- You do not offer training and education.
- You do not provide liability insurance.
- You do not market for new customers.
- You do not manage employees.

Disadvantages

- Minimal or nonexistent business growth, as you are dependent on rental income and working long hours behind the chair yourself.
- High staff turnover caused by staff moving to other salon and spa leaving for other salons and spas that offer lower rents and other perks; this in turn leads to business instability.
- The inability to manage and educate staff, and to create and promote a well-managed business with a professional, positive atmosphere.
- A lack of quality-control standards, and the damage that this can cause to your salon and spa's reputation.
- Infighting and a lack of teamwork as your salon and spa's stylists compete against each other for customers.
- Exposure to audits by state and federal taxing agencies, which are currently targeting our profession (most owners unknowingly misclassify their workers and tips; this puts you at risk for audits,

which can be triggered by anything from a labor-law issue to a staff member filing for disability or unemployment).
- The inability to sell other salon and spa services or products.

leased-space and booth-rental

The latest ownership model in which the owner contracts for a given area of space and subdivides the space into several rooms or studios, much like a doctor's office, and each room is rented to a practitioner for a service.

In both the **leased-space and booth-rental** agreements, be sure the licensed professional is given the most freedom. If you can control the products to be used, the time a person is required to work, the cost of services, and the marketing program, you no longer have a "renter" but an employee. Be sure you check the U.S. Internal Revenue Code to make sure you conform to a leased-space or booth-rental agreement. Failure could result in liability for back taxes from Social Security, violation of work-standards acts, back taxes from sales tax and income tax, and associated fines.

In summary, deciding the form of ownership that best suits your business venture should be done only after careful consideration. Use your key advisers to assist you in the process.

NAMING A SALON AND SPA

Naming your salon and spa can be tough. The hours of agony, the battles with your partners, significant other, employees, or strangers on the street—all are a part of what you may experience in developing a name. Let us simplify it for you.

The most common way people will find you online is by searching for your name. So, you have to rank in search engines for the name of your salon and spa. What does that mean?

Your name has to be easy to spell and short enough so that people can remember the whole thing. You really want the ".com" domain, and it must match your name.

It should clearly identify the salon and spa, barbershop, health spa, manicuring shop, or haircutting shop from other businesses.

Example:
Avalon Salon and Spa – *good*
Avalon – *poor* (does not tell the type of business)

It should be short and memorable.

Example:
La Dolce Vita Salon – *good*
Jake and Ann's Tonsorial Parlor for Upscale Male Hair Styling Services – *poor*

It should not be so trendy that it becomes dated when styles change.

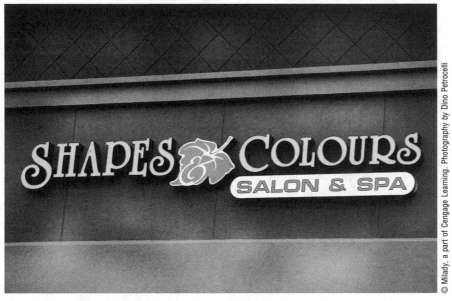

Exterior Signage, Shapes & Colours Salon and Spa.

Example:
Avante Hair Salon That "Rocks" – *poor*
Avante Hair Trends – *good*

In the end, take heart; whatever the name of your salon and spa, it is not the syllables that make it up, but the experience of your salon and spa that gives the name meaning.

Chapter 1 Summary

- Each state has its own laws, rules, and regulations for ownership of a salon and spa.

- Should a salon and spa offer services that are not licensed by the state board of cosmetology, technicians need to be licensed by another state agency and conform to their rules and regulations.

- There are generally five types of salons and spas:

  1. Hotel salons and spas

  2. Department store and fitness center salons and spas

  3. Shopping center salons and spas

  4. Freestanding salons and spas

  5. Medical spas

- Salons and spas can vary in type of ownership. The different types of ownership include sole proprietorships, partnerships, corporations, franchises, employee-owned corporations, and leased-space and booth-rental arrangements.

- The corporation style of ownership offers the owners the greatest amount of financial security against lawsuits.

- Franchised salons allow for easier startup because procedures and requirements are already in place regarding how the salon and spa should operate, all products are purchased from the franchise main supply depot allow for easier startup because procedures and requirements are already in place regarding how the salon and spa should operate, and they are supported by a larger, experienced organization, but they allow the least decision-making power to the owner.

- When naming your salon and spa, your name should identify what your place of business offers, should be easy to spell, and should be short enough that people can remember it.

Review Questions

1. List three ways in which salons and spas have changed over the years.

2. What are the three differences between a hotel salon and spa and a mall/department store salon and spa?

3. Compare sole proprietorships and partnerships. Describe one way in which they are similar and one way in which they are different.

4. This chapter referenced several potential obstacles a salon and spa owner might face with a leased-space/spa cooperative. If you were the owner, what kind of actions would you take to ensure success in your business? Consider the advantages and disadvantages provided in the text when considering your answer.

5. Why is it important that the name of your salon and spa is easy to remember and spell?

Financing the New Business

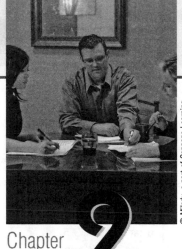

Chapter 2

INTRODUCTION

Your salon and spa businesses will require **financing** to grow. Often, lenders are very much aware that these businesses can and will struggle with the cost of varying **receivables** and high **overhead**. The success of your salon and spa is based on a local "loyal" following, and until your business has time to establish its "regulars," **revenue** can be very unstable, making it difficult to repay your **fixed loan**. The banks are well aware of this; being prepared is the answer. Most people do not have a rich relative to help finance a new project. So before you open your beauty establishment, make sure to do your **due diligence**, and fully research your options.

That being said, there are a variety of small business loan types from which to choose, and also many ways in which small business loans can be acquired. For instance, small business loans do not have to be loaned through a traditional bank, as many have been led to believe.

■ EQUITY VERSUS FINANCED CAPITAL

A few of the first financial decisions you will make are: (1) How much of your business will be **equity**? (2) How much will be financed? and (3) Should you borrow funds? Changes in the tax laws have practically eliminated the advantages of leasing equipment over borrowing capital. Look closely at all costs, add up total costs, and then see whether leasing or a loan is more affordable.

Your total cash situation will make a difference. If you are short on cash, or will need cash reserves in the foreseeable future, leasing may be the better option because you will not have to put any money down. If you

financing
Saving money and, often, lending money. How money is spent and budgeted within the business.

receivables
The amount due from individuals and companies. These are claims that are expected to be collected in cash.

overhead
Also known as *operating expenses*; an ongoing expense of operating the business.

revenue
Income that a company receives from the sale of goods and services to customers.

fixed loan
A loan in which the interest rate is guaranteed not to change for a specified period.

due diligence
An investigation of a business or person prior to signing a contract, most commonly applied to voluntary investigations. However, can also be a legal obligation.

equity
The value of an ownership interest in property, including shareholders' equity in a business.

collateral
Security pledged for the payment of a loan.

unsecured
Commonly called *signature loans* or *personal loans*. Often, these types of loans are used for smaller purchases such as office equipment/computers.

have plenty of cash, you can reduce the amount you pay each month by making a large down payment—and your total costs will be less.

SOURCES OF MONEY

It is important to understand clearly the definitions of both a *small business* and a *loan* before you jump into the process. Currently, in the United States, a *small business* is defined as an "independently" or "privately owned and operated" business that employs 100 people or fewer.

A *loan* is defined as something furnished on condition of being returned. A *small business loan*, therefore, is something furnished to a privately owned business with 100 employees or fewer that must be returned.

Business-Only Loans

Obtaining a loan can be done through the business without the use of personal credit. The business will have to justify the loan amount and have the ability to pay it back.

Business Loans

Small business loans are not always easy to obtain; banks demand **collateral**, good credit, and detailed financial reporting (including tax records and proposed planning for requested financing). The approval process for a business loan is long and may not be suitable for small businesses in need of quick financing.

Business Cash Advances

When using a business cash advance, you are not locked into a scheduled repayment plan like you are in traditional loan options. They will work with your business flow if you have a slow period by taking a smaller payment. Additionally, this will assist by providing cash in advance, quickly, without all of the red tape and strict requirements of a business loan offered by traditional banks and other lending institutions. Loans require (collateral) security, good credit, and a stable business history. In some cases, new businesses and/or businesses with bad credit may also still qualify for this type of **unsecured** business cash advance.

Small Business Administration (SBA) Business Loans

These are loans given to small businesses from private-sector lenders (banks, etc.) The SBA guarantees the loan to the bank. The SBA has funds for direct lending or loans to small businesses with long-term, fixed-rate financing for major fixed assets; this would include such items as land and buildings, but would not include paying off **reoccurring debt** such as existing credit-card debit or creating cash flow for the business.

Secured Working Capital Loans

You will find that most lenders today will require a monetary guarantee to secure a small business loan. The lenders will commonly lend you 60 to 80 percent of your collateral and will not lend you more than 100 percent of the current value. Lenders will take a **security interest** in your property and have the right to seize your collateral if payments are not received as in the terms agreed upon.

Unsecured Working Capital Loans

These are loans that are not secured by any collateral. An example of unsecured debt would be credit cards. With credit-card debt, there is nothing for them to retrieve in exchange if the loan is not being repaid. The lender is loaning you money based on your **creditworthiness**. Although it is possible, it is extremely rare to find a lender willing to give you an unsecured loan for a new business because you do not have a track record from which they can work.

Investors

Private investors are individuals who are willing to lend their money to other people. In return, private lenders receive a higher interest rate than they would get if they just put their money in the bank. Every private lender has his or her own lending criteria, which is often less strenuous than the red tape of a bank. This does not necessarily imply that getting a private loan is easy or guaranteed, just that the terms and conditions of a private loan are far more flexible because you only have to convince one person of the merits of your business proposition.

Franchise Start-Up Loans

Because they are typically nationally known and recognized, specialized financing is available to franchises.

reoccurring debt
Any debt or obligation that occurs on a continuing basis.

security interest
An interest payment used to secure the payment of a debt or obligation usually created by an agreement or in accordance to law.

creditworthiness
A creditor's measure of an individual's or company's ability to meet debt obligations.

Lines of Credit

A business line of credit is based on your business, not on you as an individual. A set amount of credit is based upon your existing inventory, which includes your accounts receivable and purchase orders, or normally up to $200,000 in business credit. This is based upon your creditworthiness with no security. This may include real estate, office furniture, or inventory.

Hard-Money Equity Loans

Hard-money loans are a specific type of asset-based loans, generally provided by private lenders or investment groups, through which a borrower receives funds secured by the value of a parcel of real estate. A hard-money loan can be provided regardless of the borrower's credit, income, or any other circumstances, with the exception of equity. Almost 100 percent of these loans are based on the equity available in the property. Different lenders have various guidelines for hard-money loans.

Construction Financing

A construction loan is any loan where the proceeds are used to finance some kind of construction. However, in the financial services industry, the term is used to describe a group of loans intended for construction and contains specifics such as interest reserves. The repayment ability may be based on the project's completion.

Residential Equity Lines

Residential equity lines are lines of credit secured by the equity of your home, which is the difference between the price for which a home could be sold (market value) and the total debts registered against it.

EQUIPMENT

Equipment Leasing

Equipment leasing is an excellent way to grow your business without significant out-of-pocket expense or having to find financing for your equipment needs, all the while obtaining tax benefits. However, in recent years, changes in the tax laws have drastically limited the advantages of leasing. Local distributors and major manufacturers often will offer leasing programs for equipment and supplies. Their interest rates may be lower than those of a bank or investors. Securing a loan from a supply dealer is often less difficult because, should the salon and spa go bankrupt, it is in a better position to repossess and resell the equipment than a bank or investors would be.

Many distributors have engineers/interior designers on staff, who will design your salon and spa for you. They will draw up a set of plans showing location of equipment, electrical outlets, plumbing, and heating systems. In most cases, if you purchase your equipment from them, this is done completely without charge. If you want only the plans, the supply house normally charges a fee for this service. One of the most valuble gifts you can give yourself is to consult your distributors. Remember, it is in their interest that your business succeeds.

Equipment Sale/Lease-Back

If you already have equipment, you can sell it and then lease back the equipment. Essentially, you are getting immediate cash for your equipment and then re-leasing it back.

Purchasing Used Equipment

Used equipment sells for 25 to 60 percent of its original value. If it suits your needs and your style, you can save a substantial sum if you buy used equipment. Be sure that this equipment is in good working order and that you have enough of each item to complete your needs. Beware of equipment that needs repair; your repair costs and the inconvenience involved may cancel out any savings. Beauty supply distributors are good sources of used equipment. They can guarantee the integrity and can loan you equipment if yours fails. If you purchase equipment directly from a salon and spa or other source, be very careful. Here are some of the problems you may encounter:

1. The equipment was not owned by the salon and spa, but was only leased, or was subject to a lien by the bank.
2. The purchase does not include all the fixtures. For example, you purchase a shampoo sink and learn that the plumbing does not go with it.
3. Is there a sales or **use tax** on the purchase? If you take it across a state line, do you need a permit, or do you have to pay another tax?

Remember to have fun! Running a small business usually involves a great deal of responsibility and can create a great deal of stress. Understanding the benefits of each type of financing will help you to make

use tax
An excise tax levied by the government on otherwise "tax-free" goods purchased by a state resident for use, storage, or consumption within that resident's state. This tax does not apply to items for resale, and is used primarily for purchases made over the Internet and on out-of-state purchases where no sales tax is applied.

the best choice for your salon and spa. Keep in mind that being prepared is always the answer. So, find the love of the game and keep playing.

Chapter 2 Summary

- One of the first financial decisions you must make is how much of the salon and spa will be equity, how much will be financed, and whether to borrow money.

- There are many sources of money that can be considered for financing. They include business-only loans, business loans, business cash advances, SBA business loans, secured working capital loans, investors, franchise start-up loans, lines of credit, hard-money equity loans, construction financing, and residential equity loans. Each has its own pros and cons, and salon and spa owners should choose the one that is the best fit for their business.

- Used equipment sells for a fraction of its original value.

Review Questions

1. Why might you choose to lease instead of paying cash when making financial decisions? Why might you choose to pay cash instead of leasing?

2. What may make a small business loan challenging to obtain? List at least two potential obstacles.

3. Describe the difference between a secured and an unsecured working capital loan.

4. Why would a private investor choose to lend his or her money to other people instead of just putting it in the bank?

5. What are two advantages of purchasing used salon equipment through a beauty-supply distributor instead of directly from a salon?

Salon and Spa Operating Costs

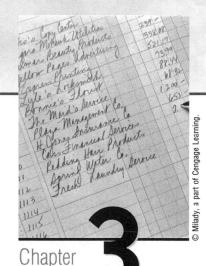

Chapter **3**

S alon and spa **operating costs** will vary according to the its location. Whether it is an elite, large salon and spa or a neighborhood salon and spa, your costs should be held to a certain percentage of the salon and spa's **gross income**. Most owners in the industry would agree that profits can run from a low of 6 percent to a high of 20-plus percent. The reason for this difference is in the definition of *profit*. If "profit" means the actual **capital gain** generated on a **capital investment** after the bills are paid, the range would be smaller. Many owners admit that some of their work is not counted as wages but as profit. Some of the areas where this occurs are maintenance, marketing, accounting, bookkeeping, delivery and pickup, and demonstrations.

Mathematically, a percentage is a ratio of two figures—that is, a fraction created by dividing one figure by a second figure.

Example:

One way to look at this is simply to figure out how much the salon and spa needs to make for the year. For instance, say you want the salon and spa to make $52,000 per year. Here are the calculations you would use to figure out what your location would need to produce per hour:

$52,000 ÷ 52 weeks in a year = $1,000 per week

$1,000 ÷ 100 hours (time the salon and spa is open each week) = $10/hr

$10/hr + a 10% profit margin = $11/hr

$11/hr = what you need to produce per hour (every hour)

Note: A fundamental way to calculate profit is

Profit = Revenue − Expenses

---

operating costs
The day-to-day expenses incurred in running the business, such as sales and administration, as opposed to production.

gross income
An individual's or business's total income before taking taxes or deductions.

profit
The positive financial gain, after all expenses have been subtracted, from an investment or business operation.

capital gain
Profit that results from selling stocks, bonds, or real estate at a price that exceeds the purchase price. The result is a financial gain for the investor.

25

capital investment
Money that is invested in the business with the expectation of income, and recovered through earnings generated by the business over several years.

gross sales
The total amount of money taken in by the salon and spa during the year; overall sales, before deducting operating expenses, cost of goods sold, payment of taxes, or any other expenses.

economic condition
A state at a particular time; "a condition (or state) of disrepair"; "the condition of finances"

wages of technicians
Wages paid to productive workers who turn out a finished product—hairstylists, manicurists, estheticians, nail-care specialists, and massage therapists.

wages of nonproducing laborers
Wages paid to employees who do not directly produce income—administrative staff, front desk associates, salon and spa managers, shampoo assistants, cleaning personnel (those who do not work on customers themselves), and repairmen (those who keep the equipment in working order).

■ SALON AND SPA EXPENSES AS A PERCENT OF GROSS SERVICE INCOME

Here are some calculations that may help in determining the actual expenses of the salon and spa; usually, two figures are given, one high and the other low. Between these extremes, any salon and spa should be represented. Profit will be determined by how well you can cut these expenses and still maintain the quality of service you wish to give your consumers. Leading salon and spa trade magazines publish yearly updates on salon and spa operating expenses and profits. You should subscribe to these and compare your own salon and spa's financial profile to that of the typical salon and spa.

Wages: 40–50 Percent

Wages should never be more than 50 percent of the **gross sales**. This figure may seem high, but let us look at what it includes. To exceed 50 percent would cause extreme management problems under any **economic conditions**.

> **Example:**
> To find the percentage cost of wages in a salon and spa, take the actual total cost of the workforce in the salon and spa (**wages of technicians**, **wages of nonproducing laborers**, taxes, insurance, records, technicians' expenses, and special events) and divide it by gross sales, and multiply by 100.
>
> $$\frac{\text{Actual total cost of workforce}}{\text{Gross sales}} \times 100 = \% \text{ wage cost}$$

1. *Wages of technicians (productive workers)*: These are productive workers who turn out a finished product. They are hairstylists, manicurists, estheticians, nail-care specialists, massage therapists, and, if you maintain a gift shop, the wages of the person in charge of this area.
2. *Wages of nonproductive laborers*: These are employees who do not *directly* produce income—administrative staff, front desk associate, salon and spa manager, shampoo assistants, cleaning personnel (those who do not work on customers themselves), and the repairman (the one who keeps the equipment in working order).
   Wages alone do not reflect the total cost of wages for the salon and spa. The total cost of wages for a salon and spa is the cost of all work paid for to anyone to whom you give a paycheck, plus all

insurance associated with the employee, including unemployment, and related employment costs.

3. *Taxes and* **licenses**: This is any form of tax paid on an employee. Social Security, unemployment insurance, federal taxes, and city "head tax" on workers—all are counted here as part of the wages of the salon and spa to its employees. Include the cost of licenses.

4. *Insurance*: Any insurance paid for employees, on their behalf, must be counted as wages. This includes life and health insurance, accident and malpractice insurance.

5. **Retirement plans**: *Such as a 401k, where an employee defers part of their current income into a tax shelter. It will then grow tax-free until the employee withdraws it. As an employer you can offer this plan with or without contributions.*

6. *Records*: Part of the cost of bookkeeping must be considered wages, because the employee is costing the bookkeeper time in making out the payroll.

7. *Technician's expense*: This includes uniforms, vacation pay, education, tickets to workshops or trade shows, health insurance, and any personal marketing such as business cards, mail-outs, and Internet marketing.

8. *Special events*: These are special dinners for employees, holiday gifts, birthday gifts, and any form of bonus paid to an employee for working in the salon and spa.

Supplies: 5–10 Percent

This is a difficult figure to calculate, since some salons and spas keep retail items and working supplies under the same heading "supply costs." Your supply bill should run between 5 and 10 percent of your gross sales. This figure depends to a large extent on how salon and spa products are purchased and the types of products used. To simplify the necessary task of tracking retail sales profitability, separate those items purchased for retail from those purchased for in-salon and spa consumption by your technicians.

To cut these costs, distributors have several ways of selling products. Plan to purchase a given item as inexpensively as possible. In some cases, an item must be purchased in quantity and stored to save money.

There are four ways to price a product, which are also the same four ways they are purchased. They are the "each" price, the "list" price, the "deal" price, and the "show" price.

1. *Each price.* The "each price" is the actual price on a unit of merchandise. Usually, this price is high in a one-unit-at-a-time sale. An example of this would be purchasing one permanent wave at a time.

license

Means "to give permission"; a license may be issued by authorities, allowing an activity that would otherwise be forbidden

retirement plan

A special savings account, such as a 401(k) or Roth IRA, where an employee either defers part of his or her current income into a tax shelter, where it will grow tax-free until the employee withdraws it, or makes contributions into the account from after-tax income, where any gains on the principal are tax-free.

2. *List price.* The "list price" is the price on a unit of merchandise where the unit represents several items. Usually, the unit consists of 12, 24, 36, 48, or 60 items, or even more. This will lower the cost because only one purchase order is made, only one delivery is made, and no odd units of merchandise are left. Usually, this price is about 10 percent less than the each price.

3. *Deal price.* The "deal price" is usually set by manufacturers to promote sales on a given item. These are specials, and to obtain them, you must purchase the merchandise during a given period. Usually, the period is from 2 weeks to a month. These items are purchased under the agreement that if you purchase a given amount, you will get an additional amount free. These free items are what decrease the effective cost of the item.

   Example:
   Purchase 24 relaxers at the list price, and the company will give you 4 relaxers free. When you figure the cost of 28 relaxers for the price of 24, you can see the savings of the deal price (about 14%).

4. *Show price.* The show price is usually applied to items sold at a dealer's show. Normally, they will sell an item at list price but will give a certain amount of another item with the show deal. This extra merchandise may or may not be the same as the original item purchased.

   Example:
   If you purchase 24 relaxers at the list price, you will receive 15 gallons of shampoo free. When you add the cost of the shampoo to the price paid for the relaxers, you can see your savings. In some cases, the show prices and the deal prices are the same.

   If you purchase in large quantities and can purchase at deal or show prices, you will automatically cut down your supply bill. To help with the storage problem, some salons and spas have worked out a system in which the distributor will store the item for the salon and spa.

   Example:
   A salon and spa purchases 240 gallons of shampoo. This is the amount of shampoo used by the salon and spa during a year's operation. The salon and spa purchases the shampoo and pays for it at the show price. The agreement is that the supply house will deliver 20 gallons of shampoo per month to the salon and spa, the remainder to be held at the supply house.

Rent: 5–15 Percent

Each salon and spa has its own **rent agreements**. In some cases, it is a flat rent; in others, it is a base amount plus a percentage of profits. If a building is being purchased as part of the business, a larger amount of rent can be paid. If the salon and spa owns the building, the rent is actually going toward paying off a mortgage, which becomes an asset to the salon and spa. The average rent paid by a salon and spa should never be over 15 percent, with the best rent being 10 percent.

Included in the rent cost should be the **property taxes** and the maintenance of items directly related to the building. If you must put an air-conditioning unit in the salon and spa and if it remains when you move, it should also be figured as rent. Additional figures should be added, such as exterior painting, decorating, snow removal, trash collection, and so forth.

rent agreement
A contractual arrangement between two parties where the landlord agrees to rent to the tenant for an agreed amount of time.

property tax
A tax that a property owner is required to pay, determined by the value of the property owned.

Cleaning and Maintenance: 2.5–4 Percent

Because different salons and spas put different items in this category, it is difficult to give an exact figure. As noted before, some salon and spa managers and owners do their own cleaning and painting. As a result, nothing will appear in this row in your budget sheet. It is quite safe to say that 2.5 to 4 percent of gross sales should cover these expenses. Included in this figure should be cleaning supplies such as soap and wax for the floor. Other items are brooms, dustpans, mops, polish, and other implements such as small electrical appliances that are used in cleaning. Included as well are toilet paper, paper towels, toilet soap, and air freshener.

Towels and Linens: About 1 Percent

This cost is again dependent upon the salon and spa's bookkeeping system. If the salon and spa does its own laundry, the cost of soap and bleach may appear low. Add to this the cost of the washing machine, dryer, and equipment maintenance, along with the cost of the towels themselves, and costs for towels and linens start to increase. Some salons and spas rent their linens. In this case, there is no equipment cost or repair, and the overall cost is just a percentage of the gross sales.

Utilities: 5 Percent

The cost of utilities is usually about 5 percent of the gross sales. This figure is sometimes included in the rent of the salon and spa. This will cover telephone, heat, lights, electricity, water, and gas. If utilities are considered part of rent costs, this row would not appear in your budget sheet.

Marketing and Promotions: 5–10 Percent

The cost of marketing should average between 5 and 10 percent during the first year of operation. Thereafter, the amount should be reduced to between 2 and 4 percent. Tracking the effectiveness of your marketing and promotions will tell you which ones should be dropped and which ones are effective, although you should distinguish between image marketing ("branding") and promotions designed to bring in business immediately. (See Chapter 8 for a full discussion on how to market.) Ultimately, what you should keep in mind is that whether it be the Internet, print material, radio, television, or another medium, all play a great part in marketing and must be considered a part of marketing costs.

Depreciation: 6–10 Percent

depreciation
A decline in the value of assets.

Depreciation is governed by tax law. As such, it can vary from time to time. The figure most commonly used is 10 percent of the purchase price. Some small items can be depreciated in one year and are included as supplies. These are clippers, brushes, combs, small appliances, and other small items.

A good accountant should be consulted about the depreciation rate and the current bookkeeping method being used by the government. A good accountant, consulted often, can save the salon and spa a good deal of time and money.

Looking at Table 3-1, you can see that a salon and spa that repeatedly spends according to the B column will run "in the red" (at a loss),

Table 3–1 Spending as a Percentage of Gross Service Income		
	Salon and Spa A	**Salon and Spa B**
Wages	40%	50%
Supplies	5%	10%
Rent	10%	15%
Cleaning and Maintenance	2.5%	4%
Towels and Linens	1%	1%
Utilities	5%	5%
Marketing and Promotions	5%	10%
Depreciation	10%	10%
Total	78.5%	105%
Profit	21.5%	−5%

whereas the salon and spa that always spends according to the A column will make a profit of 21.5 percent. Note also that in no case do we show the manager putting some of his or her money back into the business. While the figures used here are standardized, you will find a great deal of variation, both among salons and spas and within a salon and spa (among different spending categories). Cost percentages will also vary in different areas of the country.

■ SALON AND SPA RETAIL PRODUCT SALES AND EXPENSES

Again, you will find figures for the industry at large in the major salon and spa trade magazines. Compare your performance with that of the rest of the industry, and try to do better.

Example:
If you have four bottles of shampoo and sell one, you would have three left on your shelf. To find the percentage of bottles of shampoo you have sold, divide the amount sold by the whole or original number. Thus, 1 bottle of shampoo (amount sold) divided by 4 bottles of shampoo (original amount) would be the ratio 1:4 or 1/4; 1/4 = 0.25. This answer multiplied by 100 gives you the answer in percentage terms: $100 \times 0.25 = 25\%$.

$$\text{Formula}: \frac{\text{Amount sold}}{\text{Original amount}} \times 100 = \% \text{ of sales}$$

To find the percentage cost of any expense, the formula would be:

$$\frac{\text{Actual total cost}}{\text{Actual gross sales}} = \% \text{ of operations}$$

Cost of Goods Sold: 55–60 Percent

Cost of goods sold covers how much you pay for the goods you then resell to your clients. What holds back profitability?

1. *Excess inventory* (keeping more in stock than you need to). You should never run out, but neither should you have more than a two-weeks' supply on hand when your new shipment comes in.
2. *Poor retail sales performance by your staff*. Your staff should average at least 15 percent of their gross service sales in retail, and in many cases, as high as 50 percent of their gross service sales. Your

cost of goods sold
The inventory costs of those goods the business has sold during a particular period of time.

promotions should help them sell products, but they must be assertive about sales too.

3. *Poor buying habits.* If you fail to take advantage of distributors' special show prices or special promotions or, conversely, if you buy items on sale that you cannot sell, you are paying more than you have to for these items.

Supplies: 0.5 Percent

Bags and packaging, especially for such things as holiday gift packages, are a small but important expenditure. Spend the extra money to purchase packages with your salon and spa logo on them; they are excellent marketing.

Invoices and other business supplies should be purchased in 6-month to 1-year quantities in order to get the best possible price. Again, those with your salon and spa's logo on them are good marketing.

Marketing/Promotion: 2–4 Percent

Nothing sells itself. Clients need to know what is being sold and how it will benefit them. The cost of tent cards, shelf-talkers, and other salon and spa signs can be figured in here as well as the cost of samples (an excellent promotional tool) that you give away to build up business.

Commissions: 10–15 Percent

Commissions encourage sales. However, these are not necessarily paid directly to the technicians or front desk associate. Many excellent salons and spas put this money into an education fund, which they use to build their staff's skills.

Retail Sales Profits: 20–25 Percent

Retail sales profits are an important part of salon and spa income. For example, if profits from retail sales are 25 percent (an attainable figure), and if the percentage of income from retail sales equals 20 percent (also attainable), and your salon and spa brings in $250,000 in service sales a year, the resulting increase in profit to your salon and spa is $12,500 a year. If that sum is invested in a retirement plan for you, you can look forward to an earlier, more comfortable retirement than if you ignore the value of retail sales.

◦ PROJECTING A BUDGET

To project a budget using the Table 3-1, at least one figure must be known. This projection gives management the number of technicians needed and the amount of income that must be projected in order for the business to work on a sound financial basis.

The easiest figure with which to start, when thinking of opening a salon and spa, is rent. As stated before, rent is usually a flat figure until a certain amount of revenue is reached, and then an overriding percentage may be included. This flat figure is the basis on which a salon and spa must operate. Let us now project a budget for a salon and spa.

Example:
Your salon and spa will be located in a shopping center, and you have determined that the typical rent for salons and spas in such shopping centers is 10 percent, expressed as a percentage of the gross sales. You know that your salon and spa will occupy 2,100 square feet and you will be paying $15 per square foot per year. Your rent for the year is $15 × 2,100 = $31,500. Using a mathematical shortcut, you can determine what your salon and spa must gross in order to keep rent costs at 10 percent. You will need to express the percentage as a fraction of 100.

The basic formula for what you have is:

Rent ÷ Gross sales = 10/100
Invert the last figure and multiply by the rent to arrive at the gross sales.
Rent × 100/10 = Gross sales
Substituting numbers for these, we see that:
$31,500 × 100/10 = $315,000

Now you can easily calculate other costs, using percentages of gross sales based on the national figures, adjusted to your area and situation (you will have to do a little research). Change the percentages to decimal values, and multiply them by the gross sales ($315,000).

Example:

$$\text{Wages} = 50\% \text{ of } \$315,000$$
$$= 0.50 \times \$315,000$$
$$= \$157,500$$

Example:
Supplies = 5%

$$\frac{\text{Supplies}}{\$\,210,000} :: \frac{5\%}{100\%}$$

Supplies × 100% = 5% × $210,000
Supplies = $10,500

Completing the table using Salon and Spa A from Table 3-1, we find:

40% Wages	$84,000
5% Supplies	10,500
10% Rent	21,000
2.5% Cleaning and Maintenance	5,250
1% Towels and Linens	2,100
5% Utilities	10,500
5% Marketing and Promotions	10,500
10% Depreciation	21,000
Total expenses	$164,850
Total gross sales	$210,000
− Total expenses	$164,850
Gross profit *	$45,150

*Gross profit is profit before federal, state, or city taxes; licenses are usually considered a tax.

To check our figures, we go back to the formula

$$\frac{\text{Gross profit}}{\text{Gross sales}} :: \frac{21.5\%}{100\%}$$

Gross profit × 100% = Gross sales × 21.5%
Gross sales = $210,000 × 21.5%
Gross profit = $45,150

Using Salon and Spa B from Table 3-1, which has the same gross sales and floor space, and completing the table, we have:

50% Wages	$105,000
10% Supplies	21,000
15% Rent	31,500
4% Cleaning and Maintenance	8,400
1% Towels and Linens	2,100

5% Utilities	10,500
10% Marketing and Promotion	21,000
10% Depreciation	21,000
Total expenses	$220,500
Total gross sales	$210,000
− Total expenses	$220,500
Gross profit (loss)	($10,500)

This gross loss means loss to the company *before* the payment of any federal, state, or city taxes. (Licenses are usually considered a tax.) To check our figures, we go back to the formula:

$$\frac{\text{Gross loss (X)}}{\text{Gross sales}} \; :: \; \frac{-10\%}{100\%}$$

$$\text{Gross loss} \times 100\% = \$210,000 \times -5\%$$
$$\text{Gross loss} = -\$10,500$$

Analyzing the two salons and spas, we see certain things remained the same, such as utilities, depreciation, and linen. Since the salon and spa is fixed in a building, the rent cannot be changed. Changes must be made in the expenses of wages, supplies, maintenance, and marketing. While these items can be altered in Salon and Spa B, the savings would not result in a profit after taxes large enough to keep the salon and spa operating. This owner would earn a larger profit by putting the money in the bank.

HOW MANY STAFF MEMBERS DO I NEED?

Looking at the budget for Salon and Spa A, the total gross volume you must project is $210,000. The number of days a salon and spa is open per year can be computed by using 20 working days per month, using a full staff. Most salons and spas are now open six days per week; however, one technician is usually off each day, so for the purposes of calculations, a 5-day week (20 days per month) will be used. Twenty days per month times 12 months equals 240 days a year. Divide the gross sales per year ($210,000) by 240, and you arrive at a gross sales volume needed per day ($875).

The most stable service is haircutting, and most salons and spas use it as a standard to set prices of other services and time. On the average, a haircut will take about 60 minutes, which includes receiving a customer, consultation time, shampooing, doing the actual haircut and blow-dry/styling, releasing the customer, selling retail, rebooking the next appointment, suggestions, and "slip" time (should the customer be late).

Looking at a technician's service based on haircuts of an hour each and at a cost of $40 per haircut, each technician could generate $40 per hour. Since Salon and Spa A needs to generate $875 a day, you can see how many technicians must be hired to achieve your goals.

Formula: Number of technicians needed = Gross sales needed per day ÷ (Sales per hour per technician × Hours worked by each technician per day)

For Salon and Spa A:

Gross sales per day = $875

Sales per hour per technician = $40

Hours worked by each technician per day = 8

vNumber of technicians needed = $875 ÷ ($40×8)

$$= \$875 \div \$320$$
$$= 2.74 \text{ technicians}$$

$$= 3 \text{ technicians}$$ (rounding up, since you cannot have a fraction of a technician)

You now see that at least three technicians working full-time—eight hours per day, five days per week—will be needed to generate the money to accomplish the goals of Salon and Spa A. Unfortunately, this does not take into account the sick days of technicians, days off during extreme weather, fluctuation of income at certain times of the year, technicians' vacations, or a technician's leaving and moving to a salon and spa down the street. For this, go to the following formula, which works well.

Formula: Technicians needed as calculated by the steps above + 2. In the case of Salon and Spa A, 3 + 2 = 5 technicians.

Since the floor space of Salon and Spa A will comfortably hold only six to eight stations, you can see the need for securing the right technicians (with following if possible) and keeping your help happy. This will be covered further in Chapter 12, which discusses salon and spa personnel.

50% Wages	$105,000
5% Supplies	10,500
15% Rent	31,000
2.5% Cleaning and Maintenance	5,250
1% Towels and Linens	2,100
5% Utilities	10,500

5% Marketing and Promotions	10,500
10% Depreciation	21,000
Total expenses	$195,850
Total gross sales	$210,000
− Total expenses	$195,850
Gross profit	$14,150
Gross profit % = $14,150/$210,000	= 6.74%

In either Salon and Spa A or Salon and Spa B, the major expense is the wages. Wages must be low enough so a salon and spa can make a reasonable profit, yet high enough to attract and maintain good technicians. Many salons and spas have now eliminated the cleaning personnel, the front desk associate, and salon and spa bookkeepers and have reduced benefits such as vacation pay, trade show tickets, uniform requirements, and medical insurance to trim this figure.

Salon and Spa A could greatly increase its profitability by decreasing its operating costs and bringing them in line with industry averages. Let us assume that Salon and Spa A launches an aggressive cost-cutting effort, finding a more affordable space (lowering rent) and managing its equipment purchases and depreciation more effectively. We will see how that affects total profitability.

8% Rent	$16,800
6% Depreciation	$12,600
Total	$29,400
Previous rent (15%)	$31,000
Previous depreciation (10%)	$21,000
Total	$52,000
Previous profitability (1.5%)	$3,150
New profitability (8.15%)	$25,750

Profits from retail product sales should be computed separately, as stated earlier. Assuming the salon and spa makes a 25 percent profit on retail sales, a salon and spa with $210,000 in gross service income that sells even 15 percent of that in retail will bring in an extra $7,875 a year for the salon itself, while technicians and the front desk associate will receive $31,500 extra, divided among them according to their performance (assuming a 15 percent commission rate, paid directly to the person who makes the sale).

Chapter 3 Summary

- Salon and spa profits range from 6 to 20-plus percent; the range is accounted for by different definitions of profit. If profit is defined as the actual capital gain on investment after the bills are paid, the range would be smaller.

- Salon and spa expenses as a percent of gross income should be: wages, 40–50 percent; supplies, 5–10 percent; rent, 5–10 percent; cleaning and maintenance, 2.5–4 percent; towels and linens, 1 percent; utilities, 5 percent; marketing and promotions, 5–10 percent; and depreciation, 4–6 percent.

- Retail sales expense percentages are: cost of goods sold, 55–60 percent; supplies, 1–2 percent; marketing/promotion, 2–4 percent; and commissions, 10–15 percent. Total profit should be 20–25 percent.

- A budget projection gives management the number of team members needed and the amount of income that must be produced in order for the business to work.

Review Questions

1. If you wanted your salon and spa to make $78,000 per year and operate 100 hours per week, what would your location need to produce each hour?

2. What is the difference between purchasing a product at the "list" price and purchasing a product at the "deal" price?

3. What are three things that you can do to ensure a profit on the goods that you resell to your clients?

4. Why is it important to avoid paying technicians a wage that is too high? Why is it important to avoid paying technicians a wage that is too low?

Permits, Public Utilities, and Insurance

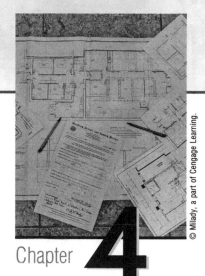

© Milady, a part of Cengage Learning.

Chapter **4**

PERMITS

At this point, we need to start thinking about obtaining licenses and permits. As the owner of the establishment, you are responsible for abiding by all local, state, and federal regulations and laws. Operating a business without a license is no different than operating a motor vehicle without a license—it is illegal! Licensing and permit requirements can vary among jurisdictions for small businesses, making it critical that your state, and local government are contacted to determine the precise documents needed for your business. Here is a list of federal, state, and local licenses along with permits you may need to acquire, prior to opening a salon and spa business.

1. *Permission from the state board of cosmetology*: This board is usually found at the state capitol or an annex thereof. Permission can be obtained by letter or in person, and upon request, the board will give you a set of salon and spa and technician rules and regulations. In some states, you receive a salon and spa license without delay. More likely, the state board will request a salon and spa plan, which shows the arrangement of the working area, the general arrangement of the supply area, toilet space, doors (interior and exterior), windows or a ventilation system, and other such information as is required by that state.
2. *Plumbing permit*: This can be obtained by your licensed plumbing contractor and will be added to his construction proposal/bill. The permit is usually obtained at the city hall in the zoning office.
3. *Electrical permit*: This can be obtained by your licensed electrical contractor and will be added to his construction proposal/bill. The permit is usually obtained at the city hall in the zoning office.

4. *Sign permit*: This can be obtained by you or a licensed sign contractor at the office of the zoning and building inspector at the city hall. Some cities are very restrictive about what size and type of signs may be displayed, especially in areas designated "historic."

5. *Building permit*: Plans showing the construction of existing walls and any new materials to be used will be necessary. You can obtain this from the architect you or the building owner hires to design your space. This, like the other permits, can be obtained from your city's zoning and building inspector. If the building site contains asbestos, it will have to be removed at considerable expense. If removal is necessary, be sure that the landlord will pay for this procedure. Also, be sure to have the building inspected for electrical wiring problems, water damage, and structural damage caused by termites or other vermin.

6. *Zoning permit*: Be sure to check on the zoning rules in the area where you intend to locate the salon and spa establishment. This is important because if the zoning is not correct for that type of business, you may have to make an appeal to have the zoning laws changed or else obtain a variance. If you have to change the zoning laws, you will have to spend much time, effort and, in some cases, money. Be sure your landlord helps to defray this cost, because it will affect his whole property. This can be done in the office of the zoning and building inspector in your city.

7. *Sales tax license*: This can be obtained from the finance department or tax commission in the city/state sales tax division. Without this license, you cannot sell any retail item in your salon and spa. A record of sales for retail must be made and kept for this department.

8. *State sales tax*: All businesses must have a sales tax number. This can be applied for from the revenue department in your state. A sales tax number is usually applied for by a bookkeeper or an accountant. Accounts for taxes on employee earnings may be set up at this time as well.

9. *Use tax*: Certain cities have a use tax on items purchased in another city and used by you to make a profit. An example is a hair dryer purchased in Denver, Colorado, to be used in Boulder, Colorado. The city of Boulder can collect a tax on that dryer in the form of a use tax. Be sure to check on use tax in your area. The information can be obtained at the city office of finance.

10. *Vending machines*: If you are going to have a candy machine, soda machine, or any other type of vending machine, you may need an additional license. Check with your local department of revenue and finance to learn if one is needed.

11. *Curbside sign permit*: Some cities will not allow signs near the street or curb area, while some do. The size and type of sign located at the end of a parking lot are quite noticeable when driving down a street. Two main items must be considered: first, a stationary design versus a revolving or moving sign statement, and second, a sign that carries a salon and spa promotion along with the salon and spa name. Check your city codes before considering a roadside sign.

■ SECURING PUBLIC UTILITIES

Securing public utilities varies from town to town and from state to state. For the most part, the plumbing, the electrical, and the building contractors will take care of the major requirements. They are the experts about size of wire, pipe, and units that will be required. They will connect you to public utilities, and all you have to do is to secure and start service.

In some places, the gas and electric companies are combined, and one stop will take care of both. You will want to know how much your service will cost per month. Sometimes an estimate will be used. If you do not already have credit with these companies, a deposit may be required. This deposit can be as much as 3 months' service. After a year of continuous service, the company will usually refund the deposit. In some cases, but not all, your deposit will earn interest. Most utilities will want your name, your address, the name and nature of the business, and three credit references.

For new accounts, the telephone company will require a deposit that will be held for 6 months to a year. This deposit is not unusual, but again, the amount of money required and the length of time the telephone company will hold it depends upon the company and its location.

There is a standard charge for phone installation, and this charge includes your name in both the white and yellow pages of the local phone directories. Each additional phone installation is an added charge, but you can purchase your own phone. You can determine many other services that your phone company offers by placing a call to the business accounts office.

Arrangements with the water company are usually taken care of by the landlord; however, it is most important that you, as a salon and spa owner, know who pays the bill. If you are responsible for paying the water bill, it is advisable to stop by the water office and apply for service about two weeks prior to opening. They, like the other utility companies, may require a deposit. The forms used are quite simple and should not take more than a few minutes to fill out.

The trash removal service is usually arranged by the salon and spa unless stated differently in the lease agreement. If it is the salon and spa's responsibility, all that is normally needed is a statement that you wish to have the service. They will ask for your name and address, the name of the business and its address, and when service should start. Some trash services furnish their own containers. If you furnish your own trash container, be sure that it meets with local and state regulations of the state board of cosmetology, the fire department, and the department of sanitation.

Environmental regulations have become very strict in many areas. Check with local authorities to be sure that your salon and spa will meet the local codes, especially regarding what is poured down the drain. Also, some states have mandated recycling programs that call for you to separate certain items from your trash and place these in different containers for collection.

The last thing you should do before moving into your salon and spa is to contact your local fire and police departments. The two departments will want to know who owns the salon and spa, where they can be reached, and when the salon and spa will be open for business. After you have your staff set up, it would be wise to give additional contacts to the fire and police departments, just in case you cannot be reached during an emergency.

 ## INSURANCE

Work with an insurance agent familiar with companies of your size and in your business. Purchase adequate coverage, but do not overspend. You can always add more as your business grows. A contract of insurance is an agreement whereby an insurance company, for a consideration called a *premium*, agrees to compensate the insured for loss or damage to the insured's property or agrees to protect the insured against legal liability. There are two general classifications of insurance: indemnity insurance and liability insurance. *Indemnity insurance* provides for payment by the insurance company to the insured for any losses suffered as a result of damage to the insured's property or person. *Liability insurance* provides protection for the insured for losses resulting from legal liability. If a person is hurt on the insured's premises and sues for damages, the insured has a legal liability.

You will be responsible for each and every person and item in your salon and spa. You will need to inquire about coverage for fire, liability, malpractice, criminal, compensation, and business interruption. If you are planning on hiring employees, you will also need **workers' compensation** insurance. Before opening your salon and spa, you will need to arrange meetings with several independent insurance agents.

These specialists write contracts for many companies, so they can select from many policies to formulate insurance for your specific needs. Compare the various proposals; by doing so, you should be able to save 10 to 15 percent of your total insurance budget.

During these meetings, have each agent provide you with insurance proposals as well as safety check sheets regarding inspection of equipment, physical structures, and protection of the public. Check insurance proposals for cancellation clauses and increased rates due to claims. See if cancellation is automatic after a number of claims have been made during a policy year. Find out if claims are honored for out-of-court as well as in-court settlements. Check the amount you will receive during the time these settlement cases or court deliberations keep you away from the salon and spa. Also ask who would pay the costs of witnesses and other related expenses.

Use the various types of insurance coverage discussed in this section as a guide to determine your specific policy needs.

workers' compensation
A form of insurance that provides compensation and medical care for employees who are injured in the course of employment, in exchange for mandatory relinquishment of the employee's right to sue his or her employer for the tort of negligence.

Types of Insurance

Fire

This type of insurance covers an individual for losses resulting from damage to property as a result of a fire. Fire insurance is a basic form of coverage that most businesses carry.

80 percent coinsurance clause: In order that the insured carries sufficient coverage to protect himself or herself from a partial loss, a coinsurance clause (usually 80 percent) has become a standard feature of most fire insurance policies. This clause makes it mandatory that the insured carries at least 80 percent of the value of the property in insurance. The failure to carry this amount of insurance automatically makes the insured a coinsurer for any partial losses.

Liability

This covers a person who has an accident on your property or the space for which you are responsible. Accidents happen when people slip on an icy sidewalk or a wet floor. The cost of this type of insurance is reasonable considering the broad span of coverage offered.

Malpractice

This protects the salon and spa and technicians against the cost of defending lawsuits, investigations and settlements, and bonds or judgments required during an appeal procedure, for instance as a result of injury due to neglect or misuse of a product while a service is being rendered. The cost of this insurance varies as you increase the number of employees in the salon and spa and the services that the salon and spa performs.

Equipment and Supply

This covers damage, other than normal wear and tear, to everything in the salon and spa.

> **Example:**
> The salon and spa is broken into, and vandalism occurs, resulting in mirrors being broken, chairs ripped, and supplies dumped. The resulting loss would be covered. The cost of such insurance varies with location, value of equipment at time of policy renewal, and various other clauses the owner wishes to insert.

Criminal: Theft, Burglary, and Robbery

No matter how family-oriented you feel your business may be or how tight security in your workplace is, theft and malicious damage are always possibilities. While the dangers associated with hacking, vandalism, and general theft are obvious, employee theft is more common than most business owners think. Here are three types of insurance that indemnify the insured for losses resulting from a criminal act:

> *Theft insurance*: Losses resulting from the disappearance of valuables or money
>
> *Burglary insurance*: Losses resulting as a result of forced, illegal entry into the premises when they are closed
>
> *Robbery insurance*: Losses resulting from the use of force or the threat of force

Workers' Compensation

Most states have enacted legislation to provide for coverage of employees who are injured as a result of accidents in the course of employment. In most states, this coverage is mandatory, and anyone who employs people is legally obligated to carry it.

Business Interruption

This form of insurance can be written as a separate policy or added to some other form of insurance, such as fire or equipment and supply

insurance. It is written to cover anticipated losses due to the interruption of business as a result of fire or some other catastrophe. Employees' loss of income can also be covered so that employees do not desert the employer while business is interrupted.

Health

This is sometimes offered as a benefit to individuals in the salon and spa under a group plan. The salon and spa may or may not pay a part of the premium. Currently, this is a very hot topic in our country. Generally speaking, the salon and spa industry has a large number of young people just "leaving the nest"—in other words, their parents' home. Health insurance can be a great point of difference when they are choosing employment opportunities.

FICA (Social Security)

All salons and spas are required to withhold **FICA** taxes from an employee's wages. For information on FICA rules and regulations, contact the Internal Revenue Service (IRS). Your accountant can do this for you and fill out the necessary forms.

FICA
Payroll taxes for Social Security benefits collected under the authority of the Federal Insurance Contributions Act, or FICA.

Loss of Income (Disability)

This insurance covers the wages of technicians in case of accident and/or illness. Usually, the salon and spa does not cover employees in this area but leaves this coverage to the individual employee to handle privately.

Life

Life insurance is most important in a partnership but is needed in all ownership types. If Partner A dies, his or her estate can freeze assets and bank accounts until the estate of Partner A is settled. Life insurance made out to Partner B will allow Partner B to purchase the partner's ownership from the estate of Partner A without Partner B having to take out a loan or being forced to sell the business to a third party after a loss.

Chapter 4 Summary

- A number of permits must be obtained before a salon and spa can be opened.
- Plumbing, electrical, and building contractors can connect you to public utilities; you will need to arrange for service to start.
- Prospective salon and spa owners should find out about both indemnity and liability insurance from several independent insurance agents.

Review Questions

1. List at least two things for which you should be prepared when you apply for a building permit.

2. Why is a sales tax license important?

3. List at least three public utilities needed in a salon and spa and the most common ways to secure them.

4. What should you ask each insurance agent you interview regarding an insurance proposal? List at least four questions.

5. What is the difference between liability and malpractice insurance?

Types of Leases and Rent Agreements

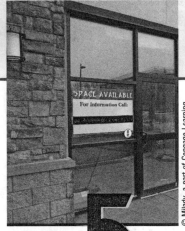

Chapter **5**

BASIC INCLUSIONS

Rent agreements are as simple or as complex as the owner of the property and the renter wish to make them. Complex or simple, they all have certain things in common. They all clearly state the name of the owner and the lessee. All leases state the location of the property to be leased, a description thereof, and for what purpose the property is to be used. Rents are stated as yearly or monthly rates, or as a yearly rate with a **percentage clause**. The percentage clause means that, after the salon and spa grosses a certain amount of business, the rent will be computed on a percentage of the gross rather than the flat rent fee. Last, all leases contain the signature of both parties and that of a **notary public**.

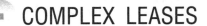 COMPLEX LEASES

Several other items may appear in more complex leases. These should be carefully read and, if questions arise, discussed with your attorney. Some other items that might be found in a lease are explained in the section that follows:

1. *Returning-the-property clause*: This generally states that you, as lessee, will return the property to its original condition or better when you vacate the property. In some cases, it will state that any improvements that you add must be left intact and in good working order. However, if a salon and spa should do any or all of its "finish out" work or improve/upgrade the property, a lower rent should be requested to offset this expense.

percentage clause
A rent arrangement in which, after the salon and spa grosses a certain amount of business, the rent will be computed on a percentage of the gross sales.

notary public
A public officer constituted by law to serve the public in noncontentious matters usually concerned with estates, deeds, powers-of-attorney, and foreign and international business.

47

2. *NNN charges*: A shopping center environment will include a **"triple net" (NNN) charge**. NNN = Common area maintenance + Insurance for the shopping center + Real estate taxes for the shopping center. *Common area maintenance* will consist of all the expenses and services for all tenants who share a common exterior of the property, such as trash, water, window cleaning, exterior lighting, and so forth. *Insurance* will be the insurance the landlord needs for the shopping center as a whole. This does not include your business insurance that you will need to operate a business. Your business insurance is separate, and when obtaining it, you will likely have to name the landlord or his lender as an additional insured on your policy. Most insurance companies will do this for a small additional charge. *Real estate taxes* are the taxes charged to the landlord by a municipality based on their system of value of the shopping center. Taxing authorities can be city, county, school systems, college districts, and so forth. All your NNN will be combined and be prorated based on the percentage of space you rent within the center. An annual amount will be calculated by the landlord and divided into monthly amounts to be paid along with your base rent. A tip will be to see if you can negotiate a cap on NNN or a cap on annual increases. Remember, NNN charges never go down; they always go up, and you will pay these increases every year.

3. *Liability clause for the property*: The salon and spa owner, in some cases, may be responsible not only for the well-being of its clients in the salon and spa but also for the sidewalk and parking area equal to the width of his salon and spa to the street. In the case of a shopping center, it could be several hundred feet.

4. *Sublease clause*: This sometimes becomes quite a problem for a shop wishing to set up a concession and seeking rental income. Since retailing is becoming more of an asset to the beauty business, be sure to find out if you can sell beauty products, clothing, wigs, hats, and so forth on this basis. To guarantee your success in this area, make sure you get all of these types of items listed in the exclusivity or use clause of your lease.

5. *Major decorating clause*: This could state that, in some cases, you might need the permission of the owner before you can remodel your salon and spa. If the change is major, you might seek help with the financial cost, which could take the form of rent reduction. The time at which you will have an advantage to get the landlord's financial help/participation will be in the negotiation for renewing your lease.

6. *Thirty days' notice clause*: This allows the landlord to show your space to prospective tenants 30 days (sometimes 60 or 90 days)

before you terminate the lease contract. This clause also gives him or her the right to place a for-rent sign in your window 30 days before your lease runs out. This would only be enforced if you have chosen not to renew or are not in negotiations with the land-lord for renewal.

7. *Single-business or exclusive clause*: This states that you will be the only salon and spa in the shopping center or leasing area. In areas where multiple salons and spas are located, the lease may contain a clause stating how close to yours (in feet) the nearest salon and spa may be located. Sometimes, the type of salon and spa is noted in the agreement to ensure that a cut-rate salon and spa or beauty school is not located too close to a higher-priced salon and spa. Try to get an exclusive on as many services as possible to give you options as your business grows. Without exclusives, a landlord may put other businesses all around you, such as nails and massage, or even another salon and spa.

8. *Deposit clause*: This states that the landlord will hold your deposit money—usually one month's rent and possibly one month's NNN—to cover any damage to the property that is not considered normal wear and tear. Protect yourself by noting all damage and/or missing items before moving in and having the landlord sign a list of these. One recommendation is to take pictures before you move in and after you move out and include them with your list (date-stamped pictures are even better). After you have vacated the pre-mises, the landlord will wait 30 to 60 days before returning all or part of your deposit money to ensure that all debts have been paid.

9. *Property waiver*: Certain property in your salon and spa may not be yours. For example, leased equipment belongs to the company from which you lease it. A property waiver will exclude such prop-erty from seizure by the landlord and will protect you from having to pay for property you no longer have control over in the event that a dispute with the landlord escalates to seizure of property.

10. *Loss-of-use-of-property clause*: Should a location in which you have leased space for your business desire to do an extensive remo-deling project, or if local progress such as eminent domain or a road-widening project takes part of the building or parking lot, you may not have access to your salon and spa for 6 months to a year. This has a *real* effect on retention of clients and the working staff. Because of the time involved, a business could lose all the working staff and booth renters and/or space renters. This clause should contain a provision that allows for a space that is the same size or larger to be available to you as soon as remodeling is completed or during any of the processes. A lower rent should also

be requested of the landlord during this period, or possibly longer, to help get your business back to its original volume.

11. *Subleasing clause*: "Subleased space" or equipment and space (booth renters) need to be addressed. Should the "leased space" need some facility alterations (new plumbing and electrical), who selects the company that will do the work? The second part of the clause should cover whether additional rent can be obtained by the landlord should the salon and spa decide to expand or remodel during its lease term. (The actual charge would be for any work done by the landlord.)

▪ THE TENTATIVE CONTRACT

tentative contract

A contract stating that, if the space can pass zoning rules and state board of cosmetology rules and regulations, and the salon and spa can get a permit for building and redecorating, an electrical permit, a plumbing permit, a sign permit, and any other permits that may be needed in that locality, on a given date, the owner of the salon and spa will sign the lease agreement.

After the space is secured, a **tentative contract** is signed. A tentative contract is a contract stating that if the space can pass zoning rules and state board of cosmetology rules and regulations, and you can get a permit for building and redecorating, an electrical permit, a plumbing permit, a sign permit, and any other permits you may need in your locality, on a given date, you will sign the lease agreement.

▪ ARRANGING A LEASE

Arranging a lease is a four-step process. First, select a location convenient to the clientele you wish to serve. For instance, a commercial area such as a busy street in a shopping district with a grocery store and pharmacy is an area in which walk-in traffic might be found. Research the location by talking to other business owners in the area. Find out costs per square foot of other competitive shopping centers or locations near your potential space; zoning restrictions; traffic counts, visibility, demographics of the people who work, shop, or live in the area; the parking situation; security; problems during bad weather; and so forth. Get a feel for whether the area is holding steady, improving, or declining, as urban decay could conceivably overtake your salon and spa well before the lease expires.

Second, determine what businesses will help your business. A grocery store or a drugstore, for example, will have a positive influence on the traffic flow for your business. A lawyer's office or a mortuary may not. Businesses with a high volume of traffic in which people have a good feeling entering and leaving will have a positive influence. This high-volume traffic will allow you to pay a larger rent, since some of the traffic will spill into your salon and spa.

Third, for the initial meeting with your landlord, have ready all information about yourself and the business you wish to operate. This information should include a personal financial profile, your years of experience in the business, a short business plan, your educational background, an approximate opening date, the number of technicians you intend to employ, bank references, and lines of credit.

Fourth, arrange for a tentative contract and first draft of the final lease contract. Both of these should be taken to a lawyer for counsel before signing. Be sure you know how to enter the contract and all the exact do's and don'ts of the lease, as well as the consequences of breaking the lease should the need arise.

Chapter 5 Summary

- All leases state certain things: the owner's and lessee's names, the day and sometimes the time the lease begins, the day and sometimes the time the lease expires, and the location and description of the property and for what purpose the property will be used.

- Additional items may appear in more complex leases, and these should be carefully read.

- Arranging a lease is a four-step process: selecting a location, determining what businesses will help your business, showing the landlord all pertinent information about yourself, and arranging for a tentative contract and first draft of the final lease.

Review Questions

1. What are two things that you can do to ensure that your landlord returns a fair portion of your deposit after you vacate the premises? Consider the common elements of a deposit clause when thinking about your answer.

2. Why is a loss-of-use-of-property clause important for a salon and spa owner? What should a salon and spa owner be sure the clause includes?

3. How can a single-business or an exclusive clause help your salon?

4. List three things that you should consider when selecting a location for your salon and spa.

Decorating and Arranging the Salon and Spa

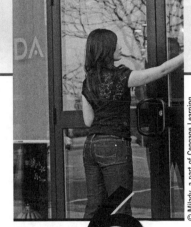

Chapter 6

This chapter deals with the physical plant of a salon and spa. Just as there are many different types of restaurants, you will find there are many different types of salons and spas also. The basic core is the same conversation, but it is your own personal creativity that will shape the specific needs of your salon and spa. First impressions are lasting impressions. But what makes a good impression? All these are questions you should ask yourself when deciding what kind of atmosphere you wish to create for your salon and spa. This chapter gives the salon and spa owner an outline of what selections are possible before making a decision.

FIRST IMPRESSIONS

Windows

Your front window, properly arranged, is one of the salon and spa's best assets. Designed effectively, displays in a shop window will increase walk-in business by as much as 50 percent. Display marketing is not new; department stores, grocery stores, and many other successful businesses spend thousands of dollars on this form of marketing. On a street or shopping mall with heavy foot traffic, window displays are necessary to attract customers.

Here are several rules to follow when decorating your windows:

1. *Windows should be cleaned regularly.* Hair spray on the inside of windows quickly clouds the glass and makes it dull. Fingerprints, tape left over from displays, and so forth create an appearance of a salon and spa not being maintained. Regular cleaning will keep the glass shining, clear, and easy to maintain.
2. *Window displays should stress one theme,* and preferably one item. It is better to have one item displayed well than a hundred items competing with each other.
3. Depending on the type of salon and spa, *promotional themes may be displayed* on the window. Another option to consider could be posters of the latest trends, or displaying the salon and spa name printed on the glass. It can be as simple as placing nothing at all in the windows, allowing the view of the salon and spa to be seen from the street, where your stylists may indeed be your best form of advertisement. Passersby can easily see the styling in progress along with any of the merchandise displayed.
4. *Displays should be changed regularly.* In this business, it is suggested that displays change every month or two.
5. *Promote your image in the window* to entice walk-ins. Also, remember the powerful lure of the words *Free, Complimentary, Gift,* and so on. Your window is your most valuable tool for luring walk-in clients who may then become regular visitors.

The Main Entrance

Your main entrance is almost as important as your window. In most cases, the entrance should contain the name of the salon and spa, leaving the window for display. In some cases, all entrances in the area are the same. Regardless of this, yours can be decorated to make it different.

All entrances should have the following characteristics:

1. They should look appealing.
2. They should be clean and well-kept.
3. They should be easy for the client to open.
4. They must be wide enough for a wheelchair to pass through without undue stress.
5. If possible, they should swing in and out. Some cities have a fire law that states that all business establishments must have doors that swing out. Check your local fire code.

6. If they are glass, they should be made of shatterproof glass, with a design on the doors to help prevent people from walking into them.

■ SALON AND SPA WALLS

Salon and spa walls can be of almost any type. They can be painted, paneled, bricked, papered, or almost any other composition you desire. Walls should be easy to clean and maintain.

The washability of all surfaces used on your walls is of prime importance. When using paint, a good-quality, long-wearing, washable paint should be used. Due to the amount of hair spray and various chemicals that collect on salon and spa walls, the extra money spent for high-quality paint is well spent. Discuss your needs with a reputable paint dealer, and remember that skimping on this point is not a savings.

The color of your walls and decorations affects your salon and spa's atmosphere. A good interior designer can help in this regard. A few simple rules follow:

- To make a room appear larger, paint it white or a light color.
- To make a long room look shorter and squarer, paint one or two of the smaller walls a darker color. An accent color on one of the walls, with the other wall white, will also make that wall appear closer.
- If a room has a low ceiling, paint or decorate the walls with vertical stripes. This will make the walls or ceiling appear higher.
- If you wish to cut down the height of a room, decorate it with horizontal lines and pictures.

Should you decide to paint your salon and spa, paint the walls with a high-grade, washable paint. This will enable you to clean more easily when needed. For the top part of the wall, you can use a water-based paint and save money. If you wish to use two types of paint, separate the two areas with a bench rail. You will never see that the paint is different.

White paint and white ceilings will make your salon and spa appear clean and light. Always keep in mind that there are design companies, interior designers, and old-fashioned personal research that can support you in color choices.

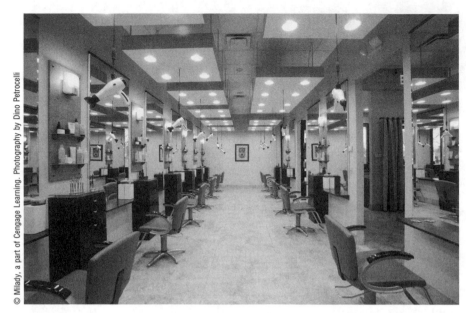

The color of your walls and decorations affects your salon and spa's atmosphere.

If you use wallpaper, make it blend with the basic color of the salon and spa. A small, muted pattern is much better than a bold one, since it will not dominate the room in which it is placed. A picture placed on a boldly papered wall will lose its effect, and so will any marketing display you place on that type of wall. A good rule is to "make it light, bright, but quiet."

Mirrors are a good idea for one wall of your salon and spa. They will make the salon and spa appear larger and will make any displays appear larger and more pronounced. The maintenance on this type of wall is minor. A good wiping with soap and water will keep the mirror wall looking good.

Pictures or posters of the hairstyle created in your business can be hung in a reception area and throughout the salon and spa. The styles created by your staff can be a great theme to display in the salon and spa. This can easily motivate your team, creating minor celebrity status within the salon and spa. Photos of styles done by the salon and spa are an effective advertisement for your technicians. Clients get to see the actual work of the stylist responsible for the style/cut/color. The featured stylist may see an increase in bookings. Pictures should be dusted regularly and changed frequently, and should definitely represent your salon and spa.

Caution: In large cities and shopping centers, the local fire department may have fire codes affecting such things as wallpaper and salon and spa decorations. For example, Christmas trees may have to be fireproof. Always check the fire codes before you invest money and effort in expensive wall coverings and decorations.

DISPLAYS

In your retail space, whether your displays and retail racks hang on the wall or are freestanding, be sure they are accessible to the clients. Customers should be able to pick up, touch, read, and even smell products. If the display is placed behind the front desk associate, you will lose more money in sales than you will lose to "shrinkage" (theft) when the racks are accessible.

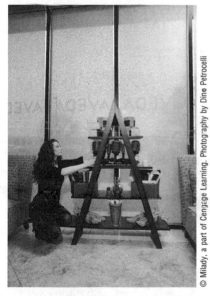

© Milady, a part of Cengage Learning. Photography by Dino Petrocelli

Be sure retail shelving is always accessible to the clients.

The stand-alone displays should be located close to the front desk associate so she or he can offer advice and answer questions. A display of inexpensively priced, eye-catching items next to the cash register will stimulate impulse buying. Of course, jewelry and small items should be kept close to the reception area, as these are prone to pilferage. If you carry expensive boutique items, these should be in a locked display case but located close to the front desk associate so she or he can show them and maintain control without having to leave the front desk.

You should be able to clean displays easily and quickly. The backdrop of the display should be easy to change and should be kept current with accent colors.

Shelves in the display section of this wall should be at least 6 inches deep, but no deeper than 8 inches. Good displays are limited to one or two major ideas. It is better to display one item well than several items poorly. Displays on a display wall should be changed frequently in order to keep your clients' interest.

Displays need to be immaculately kept, fully stocked, attractively arranged, and very well-lit. Ask your distributor for advice on setting up displays that sell products. Use your creativity and that of all your employees to make your displays as enticing and varied as possible. Observe how upscale department stores display similar items and borrow their ideas. Use seasonal themes. Above all, avoid having it look crowded or cluttered.

LIGHTING

Without planning and forethought, lighting in a salon and spa can be a problem. Five common types of lighting can be successfully adapted for salon and spa use. The type selected will depend upon salon and spa design.

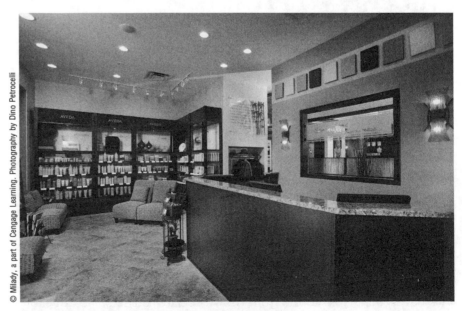

© Milady, a part of Cengage Learning. Photography by Dino Petrocelli

Without planning and forethought, lighting in a salon and spa can be a problem.

1. *Ceiling lights* are very popular. A recessed ceiling light is flush with the ceiling and will not compete with light falling on your displays; however, it will not give off much light. You will find that, if you intend to light your reception room with recessed lights, you will need quite a few of them.

2. *Spotlight or track lighting,* either recessed or suspended, can be directed on pictures and displays. This light will definitely increase sales as well as add more light to the reception area.

3. *Fluorescent tube lights* produce the most light and are the most inexpensive to operate. They do not direct your attention to any part of the reception area and are not really noticed by clients. They do very little for the décor of the room. When mirrors are present in the reception area, be sure that tubes selected give off warm tones that are flattering to the complexion. Special fluorescent lighting is now available to correct the blue or green effect of the standard tube. The new tubes give almost perfect reproduction of sunlight and can be ordered from any good lighting supplier.

4. *Chandeliers* are used for their beauty and to give light. They add a certain mood to a salon and spa that enhances the overall décor. Chandeliers should be cleaned and dusted weekly to keep them looking attractive. They should not be so large that they steal attention from displays. In selecting a chandelier, be sure that it is easy to clean. Remember, the simpler the design, the easier it will be to clean and repair.

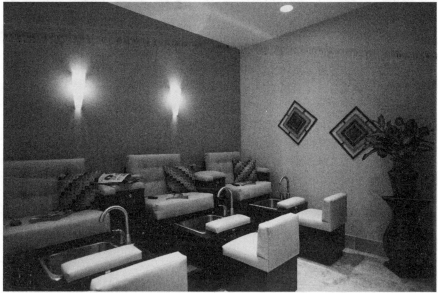

© Milady, a part of Cengage Learning. Photography by Dino Petrocell

Sconces can create atmosphere and special effects.

5. *Wall lighting* consists of two types: indirect lighting and wall sconces. Indirect lighting is usually a tube light covered by a box or panel, which directs the light toward the wall or ceiling. This type of fixture gives a soft lighting effect, but a good deal of light is lost because of the covering. If a concealed type of indirect lighting is used, and you anticipate that your clients will be reading in the area, be sure that it contains a reflector to aid in directing as much light as possible into the room. Sconces and wall lights normally do not give off much light and are used mostly as a decoration or to create special effects.

FLOOR COVERINGS

Several floor coverings can be used in a salon and spa. Floor covering is costly to replace because of the cost of labor and materials and the cost in lost business while the old flooring is being removed and new flooring laid. For this reason, choose floor covering that is durable as well as attractive and that does not limit your options for redecorating the rest of your salon and spa.

Several types of tile floors are available:

- Stained concrete

Almost every building starts out with a concrete slab. It is relatively inexpensive. There is a wide range of color and designs from which to choose. If maintained well, stained concrete can be as durable as tile, and there is no grout to deal with. However, technicians may feel discomfort when standing for long periods of time on concrete.

- Carpet

Carpet can be a real asset in certain areas. Carpet can help defer noise in a spa area; however, it would never work in a styling area. Other things to consider when looking at carpeting for your business is that some states have restrictive laws concerning carpeting in a salon and spa. Check your state board of cosmetology before you decide to carpet anything other than the waiting room.

- Hardwood flooring

Hardwood floors are now being used in salons and spas. They add beauty to the salon and spa and a source of softness to the décor. They must be sealed and treated to resist stains. New products are now on the market for this type of flooring.

- Marble

While the cost of marble tile and installation would make most salon and spa owners think twice, it cannot be denied that marble tile is quite beautiful and will definitely last as long as the salon and spa is in business.

- Rubber

The main objection to rubber tile is that it will flatten under pressure. These dents in the floor are the main problem with rubber tile. If a salon and spa has rubber tile, be sure to use an appropriate floor wax. Rubber tile can become very slick.

- Cork

Cork looks good and is fine for a den or a home, but it is too weak to last throughout the years in a salon and spa. Like wood-covered floors, cork tile will stain if not given the proper care.

- Vinyl

Vinyl is available in rolls or tiles. Vinyl can be cost-effective flooring for certain areas of your salon and spa. It is easy to install, and it comes in many colors and designs; however, if you are looking for something that is durable and long-lasting, you may want to be aware that if not installed properly, vinyl tile can fade, scrape, and lift.

- Ceramic

Ceramic tile floors are close to marble when it comes to standing up to wear. They clean up well and do not need to be polished constantly. The grouting between the tile seems to be the major problem with this type of floor. The grouting placed between the tiles of a ceramic tile floor can discolor over time. If you drop a glass bottle on a ceramic tile floor, it will break. There is no way to cut down on breakage with this kind of floor, but cleanup will be easy.

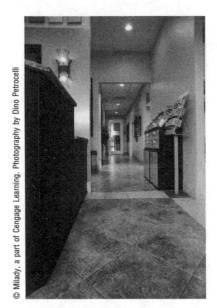

Several floor coverings can be used in a salon and spa.

Regardless of what type of floor covering you choose, it should have several important features:

- It must be stain-resistant.
- It must look good.
- It must be easy to match (in case you decide to enlarge the salon and spa and want to use your previously tiled floor).
- It should be easy to clean.
- It should not be slick when you wax or polish it.
- It should be resistant to water spots, salon and spa chemicals, and wet, muddy shoes.

As with other furnishings and design, a floor covering that is predominantly a neutral color works best.

Check the local building codes and your state board for regulations governing what types of floor covering may be used. Choose a type that can handle heavy traffic without showing wear and that is resistant to staining and the chemicals used in salons and spas.

WAITING AREA

This area will set the tone for your salon and spa. Whatever style of decorating you choose, it needs to reflect who you are and what type of clientele you wish to receive.

Chairs

These chairs should be attractive and have a certain warmth and charm to them. When purchasing waiting chairs, consider these points:

1. *They should be good-looking* and an asset to the décor of the salon and spa.
2. *They should be the correct size.* If your waiting room is small, do not overpower it with overly large waiting chairs. The chairs should be large enough for a 250-pound person, but comfortable for a small person as well.
3. *All waiting chairs should be easy to clean.* Be sure that their coverings can be cleaned with soap and water.
4. *All waiting chairs should be simple in design* and easy to move around the waiting room.
5. *Fabric-covered chairs should be long-wearing,* fireproof, and nonporous.
6. The *chairs should have good springs,* padding, and foam rubber. If you cut costs here, you will have to purchase new chairs in a few years.
7. *Chairs without arms are more comfortable* because they are less confining and cooler. With chairs that have arms, the air has no way of circulating around the customer.

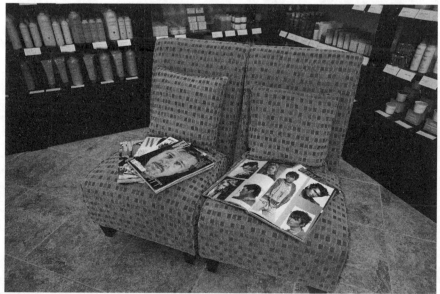

© Milady, a part of Cengage Learning. Photography by Dino Petrocelli

Chairs without arms are more comfortable.

The Coat Rack/Closet

Coat trees are impractical and unsightly when overburdened, making a coat rack preferable. A good coat rack with sturdy plastic or wooden hangers is a necessity. Be sure that the rack is out of the way but within sight of the front desk associate (for security). The best design is one that includes a rack above for hats and a rack on the sides for umbrellas.

A coat closet may be a good idea, but there are a few things to consider: first, they cost money to build, and second, when you enclose damp clothes, you are bound to create odors that will affect everyone's clothing in that area.

The best solution seems to be a compromise between a coat rack and a closet. This can be built on a stationary wall, and consists of two supports and a pole. A shelf above is a must for hats and packages carried by clients. Because this area is open at the top, no musty odors will accumulate. The area should be close to the front desk, making it easy for him or her to hang up clients' coats when they arrive. A light in that area is a must. Clothes hangers should be made of wood or sturdy plastic. These will support the weight of a winter coat as well as a sweater. Metal hangers often leave creases in heavy clothing and tend to bend and sag. Wooden hangers can be purchased at a reasonable cost and should be replaced when needed. Remember that your geographical area will determine the size of a coat closet/rack. In warmer climates, there is going to be less need for bulky coats; therefore, a smaller space is needed.

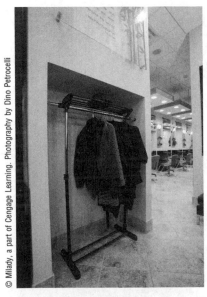

To maximize space, the coat rack can be built in.

Magazines, Books, and Newspapers

Before selecting magazines for your salon and spa, be sure to study your clients' interests. Make sure to have magazines that reflect their needs.

- Fashion
- Pop culture
- Sports
- Styling
- Entertainment

In selecting the number of magazines for your salon and spa, a general rule is "three magazines for each technician." A shop of six professionals would have 18 magazines. These magazines can be purchased by subscription at a lower price than if they were obtained at a newsstand.

Magazines should be changed frequently. No magazine should remain in the salon and spa beyond its life span. If it is torn, written on, or outdated, it is time to remove it from the salon and spa.

A few other types of reading materials you may consider having include the local newspaper and a few paperback books.

Magazines can be placed on a table or a magazine rack. They should never be left on chairs or the floor.

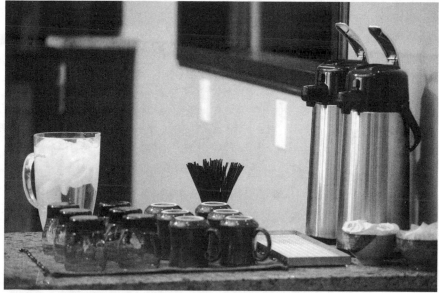

© Milady, a part of Cengage Learning. Photography by Dino Petrocelli

Most salons and spas have a refreshments table.

When magazines are no longer needed by the salon and spa, a great way to recycle them and an easy way to promote your business is by giving them to rest homes, senior centers, and hospitals.

Coffee

Most salons and spas serve coffee, tea, or other refreshments to their customers. A clean coffee container along with cups should be part of the equipment in the styling area/waiting area. If coffee is served, a small table on which to place a cup is needed. Plastic cup holders and plastic-coated cups are quite inexpensive and do a much better job than plain paper cups. You may choose to use ceramic coffee mugs as an alternative, but you will need to consider purchasing a dishwasher for sanitation reasons. Sugar and powdered creamer should also be provided. The coffee container, cream and sugar, cups, and a few spoons should be placed in a convenient place in the styling area for the use of both the clients and the technicians. Used cups should be the responsibility of the technician and should be emptied and replaced as soon as possible after use.

THE FRONT DESK

The reception or front desk is often the "nerve center" of the salon and spa and controls all its activities. A poorly organized desk will cost

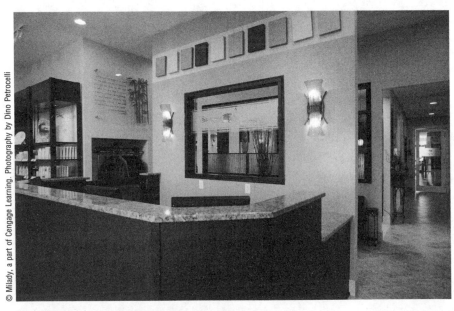

© Milady, a part of Cengage Learning. Photography by Dino Petrocelli

The "nerve center" of the salon and spa.

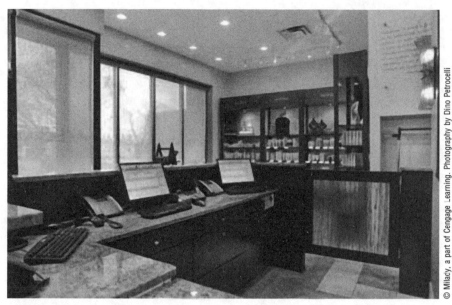

As the "nerve center" of the salon /spa, the reception desk should be well organized and clutter free.

many hours of wasted time on the part of your front desk associate and technicians. As such, it is the most important piece of furniture in the reception room. The following is merely a suggestion, not mandatory, of how a front desk might be set up.

The front desk should be about 4 feet wide and 2 feet deep. Six inches of space needs to be available for check-writing, signing credit-card receipts, and placing a purse or bag while the client pays his or her bill.

A space for the shelves and drawers can be to the right. The top drawer should be 1.5 feet wide and should be as deep as the desk. It should be divided into two sections. The first section is used as a cash drawer, and the second can be used as a safe with a key. This drawer should be 3 inches deep, and the outside of the drawer should also have a lock and key.

Desk Accessories

On the desk table, you should have:

1. *A computer.* Today, most salons and spas have computer systems, although some salons and spas may use a paper appointment book. Remember to provide adequate electrical support to the computer components with a dedicated electrical outlet and electrical breaker. The electrical outlet and breaker will prevent interruption due to

overloaded lines used in the styling area. An additional telephone line is needed for the computer so that the salon and spa's service lines are not overloaded. For more information on computer operation, see Chapter 7.

2. *An appointment book* that is large enough for your business and easy to flip from day to day. Make sure to use a pencil to schedule appointments, and have an eraser on hand.

3. *A telephone.* This is usually placed on the left side of the desk so the front desk associate can hold it with his or her left hand and write with his or her right hand. A telephone mounted on the side of the desk is better. This will keep it out of the way. An added convenience for the busy front desk associate is a headset-type telephone that will allow free use of both hands while answering the phone. Though not inexpensive, such a phone accessory will prevent stiff neck muscles and dropped phones that can occur otherwise and will allow the front desk associate to work more quickly.

4. *A container with several pens and pencils.* Pencils and pens have a habit of walking away with your customers. Those having your salon and spa name on them may be great marketing items.

5. *A calculator.*

6. *A box of appointment cards.* An appointment card should be given to each client as he or she leaves the salon and spa.

7. *A message pad* for notes and messages should be available at all times.

8. *A menu/price list* may be placed on the top of the desk table for easy access by clients.

9. *A client's service ticket holder/folder* should be placed at the very rear of the desk and out of the way of conducting business.

Remember: Less is better when it comes to clutter.

If you do not have an office, the front desk can house your copies of operations material, such as:

- Job application forms
- Interview sheets
- Technician evaluation sheets
- Technician check sheets
- Technician daily report sheets
- Public-relations file
- Supply company's files
- Inventory report forms
- Supply order forms

Note: If your salon and spa is computerized, the forms will be found in the computer, and it may be necessary to have only a few hard-copy items, such as job applications, held at your front desk for easy access. Please refer to Chapter 7 for more information.

THE STYLING AREA

Selecting the décor for the styling area is one of the core decisions you will make in your new salon and spa. It should be in the same general style and mood as the reception room (which could be in the same structural area), but if you choose to depart from the style of the reception area, be sure that there is a transition area between styles. The styling area consists of:

- Styling chairs
- Styling stations
- Shampoo bowls
- Dryer chairs
- Station/bar for styling, tinting, or special services
- Manicuring tables
- Pedicure spa chairs

The way you arrange them will give your salon and spa a definite personality, but be careful that you allow sufficient room to work and that traffic can flow smoothly through your salon and spa. Following are discussions of two distinct types of styling stations as well as other equipment you will need to examine as you choose what is the best suited for your business.

Wet Stations

Wet stations are basically "all-in-one" stations, designed to perform both wet and dry services, which are built by companies specializing in salon and spa equipment. Typically, stations are 5 feet per section and are placed on a wall. The sinks are usually in the center and are about 20 inches to 2 feet in width. On each side of the sink, there is generally cabinet space. These cabinets hold clean towels, clean combs and brushes, a soiled-towel hamper, and a miscellaneous shelf. The top of this cabinet is often used to hold a normal supply of hair-setting preparations for the technician. In the back of the sink is the normal place to house the shampoos and conditioners.

Wet stations are ideal for chemical services. Since these are often best located separately from the basic styling/cutting station, you can save money on the plumbing installation by grouping the wet stations and designating these as chemical-service stations.

Advantages

- No time is wasted taking the client to and from the shampoo bowl.
- Once the client is seated, he or she does not have to be moved. This is an important advantage for clients in wheelchairs.
- Each technician is responsible for the cleanliness of his or her own station as well as restocking supplies (refilling shampoo bottles etc.).
- The client can be kept at the sink as long as necessary without interfering with other clients.
- Shampoo chairs (converted styling chairs) can be raised or lowered to conform to the client.

Disadvantages

- The cost of installation is greater (the added plumbing needed for the station).
- The styling area is less flexible.
- Wet stations require more products to be placed on them (e.g., shampoos and conditioners) than a dry station would involve.
- Wet stations can take up more floor space than many styles of dry styling stations.
- Styling chairs are sometimes uncomfortable when in the shampooing position.

The sink portion of the wet station is generally covered when not in use, giving the technician added counter space. When the sink is being used, the top of this section is either lifted or slid to one side, leaving the sink open for use. If the stations are closer than 5 feet (the center of one sink to the center of the second sink), technicians will be bumping into one another. The sinks should be from 2.5 to 3 feet from the floor. The chairs used for shampooing and styling should be close enough to the sink to let the client's head rest in the sink comfortably.

Mirrors in a wet styling section may or may not extend the length of the station. Regardless of the size of the mirror, it should be kept clean and neat.

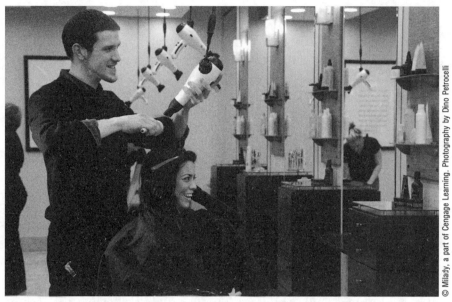

Selecting the décor for the styling area is one of the core decisions.

Dry Stations

A dry station can be used as a styling station or a chemical station. The main difference is that this station does not have a sink in it. While the wet station will extend 7 feet out from the wall for ultimate comfort (this includes the styling chair), the dry station and styling chair will extend out from the wall no more than 4 feet for ultimate comfort. The chairs in a dry station should be on a 5-foot center. Placing them closer cramps the technicians.

Advantages

- The principal advantage in this type of arrangement is that it makes servicing multiple clients easy. While one client is being shampooed by an assistant, you may be working on another client.
- The initial cost of plumbing could be drastically different; with one room as a central shampooing area, your plumbing cost would be less than having plumbing at every station.
- Mirrors can be placed so that both shorter and taller clients can easily see themselves. The styling chairs should be able to compensate for this difference in height between different clients.

Electrical Outlets in Styling Stations

With curling irons, flat irons, and blow dryers, additional wiring is needed. Each station should have electricity to support two irons and an 1,875-watt blow dryer. Since some stations are also equipped with ultraviolet sanitizers, clippers, and other electrical equipment, each station should be separately wired. A good electrical contractor can do this at a reasonable additional cost when the salon and spa is established; rewiring later can be costly—in some cases, up to four times as much as the original cost. Put each station on a separate fuse or breaker switch so that overloading will not be a problem. For additional security, these switches can be turned off at night, preventing a fire caused by overheated curling irons or faulty appliances left on overnight.

Styling Chairs

The styling chair is as important to the client as it is to the technician. It should provide full comfort to the client while allowing the technician complete freedom of movement. If it is to double as a shampoo chair for wet stations, it should be able to be released into the shampoo position from either side of the chair. The lock should be easy to work and should hold securely when the chair is in the lowered position.

All styling chairs should be covered in washable, stain-proof coverings that are easy to keep clean. Chairs with open arms are cooler and easier to care for than bucket-type chairs, and they also prevent pins, combs, change, and dust from collecting between the sides and bottom. A foot bar or a foot rest adds to the client's comfort.

Hydraulic chairs should be able to be raised 11 inches with a foot lift. They should never be placed closer than 5 feet from center to center; to do so would cause the technicians to bump into each other as they work.

Separate release pedals are usually hard to reach with the foot and present another item to be maintained. Hydraulic fluid and working parts should be easily accessible for maintenance and repair. Electric hydraulic chairs are not always worth the extra money. The main disadvantage is the electrical cord, which must be recessed in order to prevent the technician from stepping on it.

Styling chairs are designed for people who are 5'2" in height. The lifting system allows the chair to increase in height by 6 inches, so a person who is less than 5'8" tall can work well with this styling chair. For people who are over 5'10", a slight modification can be made. Remove the shank at the bottom of the seat of the styling chair. Take the shank to the machine shop and have the machinist make a shank that is 6 inches longer. The styling chair with the new shank is great for people up to 6 feet tall. The new styling chair will be slightly higher when in a down position, but will save a stylist from having back problems in a few years.

Dryer Chairs

Traditional dryer chairs are usually 2.5 feet from the back to the front, including the dryer hood. They are 2 feet wide, and the seats are from 18 to 20 inches from the floor. A foot rest may or may not be attached, and this could extend the chair to 4 feet from the back of the dryer to the end of the foot rest. These chairs should be the most comfortable in the entire salon and spa. The client may sit in them anywhere from 30 minutes to an hour or more.

They should be easy to clean and maintain. The covering of this chair should be of leather, synthetic leather, or a good-quality plastic. Fabrics can be used, but cleaning can be a problem. In most cases, the dryer and dryer chair are in one unit, but this does not always have to be the case. The chair can be separate, and the dryer may remain free. Dryers can be attached to the wall or ceiling and, because of their extendable arms, any chair can be used for drying purposes.

A dryer chair should have the following features:

1. It should be comfortable.
2. It should be large enough to seat a heavy person yet small enough to make a small person feel comfortable.
3. It should be able to be cleaned quickly and easily.

All dryers, whether connected to the chairs or not, should have the following features:

1. They should come apart easily for quick cleaning.
2. They should be grounded adequately to prevent shocks.
3. They should have a temperature control that is easy to reach by both the client and the technician.
4. They should be able to be lowered or raised with one hand by either the client or technician.
5. They should have an automatic cutoff if the dryer gets too hot.

Note: Today, more hairstyles are being finished out with a blow dryer and hot iron than with a dryer station.

Manicuring Tables

Manicuring tables are important in the salon and spa. They should be about 2.5 feet high. The height of a manicure table should be such that a client's arm and hand comfort is maintained during a manicure. These tables should be covered with a nonporous top, preferably Formica or plastic, and should be kept clean at all times. The table should have sufficient light for the technician to give a good manicure. The light should be on the right of the table and should illuminate the working area but should not be strong enough to irritate the patron's eyes. Below the top of the manicuring table should be a drawer to hold the technician's manicuring tools. (Check your state board for regulations covering the care of tools stored in the manicuring drawer.) A stool for the technician should be available. This stool should be able to be raised or lowered as the technician wishes. Casters on the stool and table will allow them to be moved at will by the technician.

Because of health hazards posed by some of the chemicals and materials used in nail services, special precautions must be taken. A separate area for nail stations is by far the best option. The nail stations themselves should each have its own **Ventilation system** to vent noxious fumes and dust outside. Although some nail stations have filters and seem to be more advantageous because they require no outside venting, remember that filters quickly lose their effectiveness. Also, some filters remove odors but not the hazard.

ventilation system
The process of "changing" or replacing air in any space. Often used as a device to control the temperature or remove moisture, odors, smoke, heat, dust, and so forth. Ventilation includes both the exchange of air to the outside as well as circulation of air within the business.

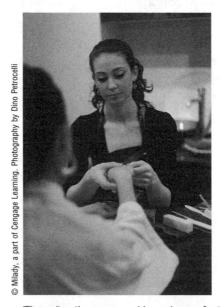

© Milady, a part of Cengage Learning. Photography by Dino Petrocelli

The client's arm and hand comfort should be maintained during a manicure.

You should check with your state board and local environmental authorities to see what precautions are mandated by law, but remember that we live in a litigation-prone society. You may adhere to all regulations and still be sued 10 years later by an ill employee because you did not take all precautions that were available—a sobering thought.

Another serious consideration is sterilization of equipment. In part because of the real risk of transmitting potentially fatal diseases and in part because of bad publicity generated by unregulated nail salons and spas that do poor work in unsanitary conditions, manicurists and pedicurists must overcome a negative image. State boards often require basic sterilization procedures. These must be followed scrupulously. Salon and spa owners who want to build their nail business must be sure that the clients are constantly assured that good hygiene is being practiced and that the work is of the highest quality.

In addition to manicures, pedicures have become a popular service in the salon and spa. A pedicure chair with a foot bath and running water needs to be connected to both the water supply (hot and cold) and a drain. Some states allow flexible water connections such as a hose found on a clothes washer with a discharge hose connected to a drain. Before purchasing, check with the state board of cosmetology for their requirements and the local plumbing codes to satisfy all their requirements, regulations, and laws. An automatic shutoff is a good idea to keep the foot bath from running over or in case of an electrical short. Most clients find no problem stepping up to this chair; however, older clients may still need to have a pedicure done in a styling chair, dryer chair, or waiting chair. This requires a pedicure stool that can be placed out of the way and stored when not in use. The rollers on these stools should have a "lockdown" attachment prohibiting them from moving while a client is receiving service.

■ PURCHASING FURNITURE OR EQUIPMENT FROM A DISTRIBUTOR

Although you can purchase salon and spa equipment and furniture directly from a manufacturer or (used) from another salon and spa, going through a distributor offers certain advantages.

1. The dealer will often give you free help with design in exchange for purchasing equipment from his or her company.
2. Distributors will usually help out with "loaners" when equipment goes bad.
3. Distributors will often pick up defective merchandise rather than your having to make the arrangements to ship it back to the manufacturer.

Chapter 6 Summary

- The reception area is seen first by a client and makes the strongest impression.
- A carefully arranged display area will increase the sales of cosmetics, beauty supplies, grooming products, styling aids, styling equipment, and retail products.
- No magazine should remain in the salon and spa beyond its life span. If it is torn, written on, or outdated, it is time to remove it from the salon and spa.
- Walls should be easy to clean and maintain; floor coverings should be durable.
- Wet stations cost more to install than dry stations, but have their advantages.
- Both styling and dryer chairs should be chosen with the client's comfort in mind.
- Purchasing equipment from a dealer offers certain advantages.

Review Questions

1. What are at least three things that a salon and spa owner can do with windows that will encourage customers to come in?
2. Where should retail racks be located? Why?
3. Why might you choose fluorescent tube lights instead of chandeliers in your salon and spa?
4. What should you remember regarding magazines for your salon and spa? List at least four considerations.
5. List three advantages of wet stations compared to dry stations.

Salon and Spa
Business Tools

Chapter **7**

A salon and spa that is conceived on paper and developed with wood, textiles, stone, water, and electricity will eventually become a living establishment. Salons and spas, like people, have personalities. The personality is formed in the same way that a person's personality is formed. Personality is dependent upon original composition (actual materials), the brains (management), the working parts or organs (technicians), the support systems (supplies and maintenance), and, finally, the work it produces. A salon and spa, like any working unit, only functions well when all parts are in good working condition.

A salon and spa that is functioning well can be said to have a good personality. A salon and spa personality is governed by five main components. If any one of these breaks down or is not used, the salon and spa will suffer. They are:

1. The original composition
2. **The management**.
3. The staff members
4. The support systems
5. **The inventory/supplies**

All the parts must function well, or the salon and spa will fall into trouble. If the trouble is not corrected, the salon and spa will cease to exist.

management
The person or people who perform the act(s) of management: getting people to work together to accomplish desired goals and objectives efficiently and effectively.

ORIGINAL COMPOSITION

Regardless of how the salon and spa is started, or who owns it, it must be well-built. Some of the most important things to check when purchasing or starting a new salon and spa are:

1. *Walls, floor, and ceiling.* All of these must be easy to maintain. They must be sturdy and not need constant repair.

   Example:
   A salon and spa whose ceiling is cracked and has plaster coming loose will not reflect well on its owners or managers. The floor should be replaced before it completely wears out and becomes decomposed. The walls should be constantly maintained. Chipped paint, dirty wallpaper, or loose wooden panels all give a salon and spa a bad image.

2. *Plumbing and electrical connections.* These should be checked and maintained at least once a month, and repairs should be made when needed. Plumbing drains and pipes should be cleaned with a good pipe-and-drain solvent. This solvent should keep the plumbing free from hair and other buildup. Hot and cold water taps should be checked for leaks, and faucet washers should be replaced as needed. Shampoo hoses should be changed when worn out. Electrical outlets and lights should be constantly checked and replaced when needed. Burned-out lights indicate neglect.

3. *Brushes, combs, and manicuring equipment.* These must be constantly replaced and always be in perfect condition.

4. *Towels, robes, and so forth.* These should be replaced as needed and kept extremely clean.

MANAGEMENT

Management, the brains of the salon and spa, must make the decisions and motivate the workforce. Here is a brief summary of what the salon and spa management (owners and managers) must do in order to perform well.

1. *Attend to the needs of all parts of the salon and spa.* From the physical condition of the salon and spa to the nuances of psychology, the responsibility for observing these and reacting to them falls on the management. They work together as a whole, and thus none can be neglected without detriment to the others.

2. *Help the staff succeed.* By helping each staff member succeed, the management builds a strong, loyal staff. Also, the salon and spa's success depends on the success of each person working in it.

3. *Allow the staff to participate.* Nothing will build up resentment among employees in any business more rapidly than feeling that

they have no voice in their own future. Allowing people a voice, at least in an advisory capacity, builds each person's sense of worth, and that is important to good performance and good relationships. Also, employees really do have information that is valuable to contribute. While the management retains control over final decision-making, by tapping the various resources among the staff, they will find that the whole is truly greater than the sum of its parts.

4. *Develop your own management skills.* Management is not easy, but education makes it less difficult. Invest in management training. You will find many answers there, and also others with whom to share your feelings and on whom you may call for an objective voice during difficult times. Remember, "The speed of the leader is the speed of the team."

■ STAFF MEMBERS

It takes time and money to select the right employees. Too often, employees seem to function well alone, but do not, or will not, function with one another. Helping your employees work together is called *teamwork*. It is your job as a salon and spa owner and manager to coordinate your staff to work as a team in your salon and spa. No good salon and spa has technicians working only in pairs, or by themselves. It must be a team effort. Here are a few ways in which you can develop salon and spa spirit:

1. *Technician thanh-you.* It is interesting that a new technician is the one who receives the most 'attention, while the steady, hardworking, durable employees seem to be forgotten. When a new employee is hired, the employer may be spending anywhere from $3,000 or more to get him or her started. This figure includes guaranteed salaries, marketing, and special promotions. After an employee has been with the business for three to five years, he or she is actually making money for the salon and spa. Instead of being praised for his or her efforts and the time the employee has worked for the firm, he or she is often taken for granted.

   Spend a few dollars occasionally on gifts for your technicians to let them know how much you appreciate their work. A dinner party will do the same thing. Honest praise is a valuable management tool; use it.

2. *Help all you can in the salon and spa.* Cooperation is contagious. Helping with a shampoo here or seating and draping for another stylist will get many extra dollars' worth of effort out of your technician. When you are making a decision about the salon and spa, ask the employees to help you; whether you take their advice or not makes no difference—they still like to be asked.

3. *Above all, teach them.* There are only three ways technicians can increase their income in this industry, and ultimately that is what will keep your staff happy with you for any length of time:

A. Increase the average ticket in both service and retail. Teach them to *educate* the client, not *sell* the client. A "no" only means "I don't have enough information."

B. Increase the number of times the client sees you in a given period of time. Teach them how to rebook; this is known as the customer "turn." It is the number of times they comes to see you in a year.

C. Increase the number of clients you see. Teach them to ask for referrals and market themselves in their everyday life.

▪ SUPPORT SYSTEMS

Support systems include your **computer systems**, bookkeeping system, working capital, front desk associate, and maintenance department. Like food, the support system will nourish, feed, and revitalize your salon and spa. It can keep it running in a good, smooth, profitable fashion. Let us look at each of these things separately.

Computer Systems

Hardware

Hardware includes the computer, computer monitor, keyboard, mouse, speakers, printer, and auxiliary equipment.

Software

Software is computer programs that do specific jobs such as appointment management, accounting, and inventory.

Selecting a Computer Program   There are several companies whose sole business is computer programming. Remember, you are in the driver's seat when choosing a program/software that fits your business. Search for software that provides exactly what you want. If the software cannot produce it, look elsewhere. Most salon and spa software companies will provide you with numerous training opportunities for you and your staff.

Training should be done when the salon and spa is closed. Several sessions of 1 hour each are more productive than one 4- or 8-hour session. The programmer should produce a book or instruction sheet to aid in your salon and spa's education.

computer system
A programmable machine that receives input, stores and manipulates data/information, and provides output in a useful format.

hardware
An object that is tangible, such as disks, disk drives, display screens, keyboards, printers, boards, and chips.

software
The collection of computer programs and related data. This term was originally coined to contrast with the term *hardware* (meaning physical devices).

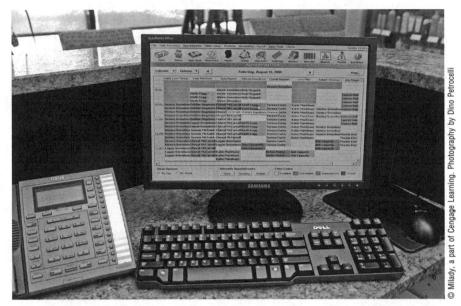

Computer programs do specific jobs such as appointment management, accounting, and inventory.

There are usually several ways to perform some of the programmed functions. Computer software companies delight in showing you all the ways to get from A to Z. Remember when you were learning to do pin curls, and the instructor showed you four ways to do them? After a few hours, you were so confused you could not do anything. The same is true here. Learn one way. As an owner, you may or may not want the front desk associate to do payroll, bank deposits, inventory, and so forth. Train the front desk associate in only those areas that are part of the job description. The complete training program should be taken by the salon and spa owner and another person, such as a husband, wife, daughter, son, or manager, so the salon and spa can continue to work effectively in the event of the owner's absence due to illness or vacation. As new front desk associates are employed, they will have to take the training, and you, as an employer, will be expected to pay for their training and salary during this time. Select your front desk associate well. Most front desk associates will leave a salon and spa's employment in three to four years.

How Many Computers Does a Salon and Spa Need?

The front desk associate must have a terminal. The salon and spa owner needs a computer in the office. The system may consist of one computer with one printer and one scanner, or one file server with two keyboards and monitors. Again, this can be designed by your computer specialist. A portable computer (laptop) or a terminal at home with a virtual private connection (VPN) to the salon and spa's computer could allow some work to be done at home when the salon and spa is closed or when the owner has a day away from the salon and spa. Think ahead. It is best to purchase everything at once so all items work together.

Internet Access

This is an item that today would be considered extremely valuable. It is not only helpful for information on products and their use, it can be used for ordering, checking prices, and finding people looking for employment. Many salons and spas today are also providing areas with wireless access, complimentary laptops, and so forth for their clients' convenience.

Bookkeeping System

If you were expecting a check on the first of the month and it did not come until the fifteenth, you would not be pleased. Your employees feel the same way about their paychecks. Be sure that the bookkeeper is prompt about paying your employees and that the checks are accurate. Nothing is worse than a late check or one that is incorrect. The booking can be done in-house or outsourced. There are several companies that provide a payroll service.

Working Capital

working capital
Current assets minus current liabilities, measuring how much in liquid assets the business currently has available to build the business. This number will be affected positively or negatively by how much debt the company is currently carrying

A salon and spa must have enough **working capital** (in cash and a checking account) to make change, cash checks, and pay bills. A front desk associate should never have to go out of the salon and spa to look for change. Also, you should have enough money to keep the business in operation for two months without having to worry about closing the salon and spa. Too often, a salon and spa has to cut down on hours because there is not enough working capital.

Front Desk Associate

Not all salons and spas have front desk associates; however, in many salons and spas today, the front desk associate is the nerve center of the salon and spa. He or she is the one who will keep the whole system running smoothly. The front desk associate's duties should be well-defined and known to everyone in the salon and spa. Knowing the job's limits of authority and responsibility, the front desk associate will be able to keep everyone happy. The front desk associate is the salon and spa's number-one public-relations officer and must reflect the best image for your salon and spa. A strain on this person can throw the whole system into a downward spin.

Maintenance Department

A salon and spa that is constantly disorderly and dirty will self-destruct. You must either hire a good maintenance person or delegate duties between staff members. This person's duties should including cleaning the windows, doors, and walls and painting them when needed; he or she should care for the restrooms, change light bulbs when needed, and so forth.

■ THE INVENTORY SUPPLY ROOM

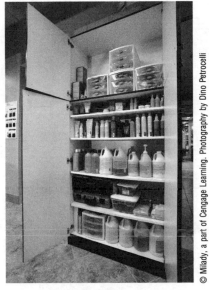

© Milady, a part of Cengage Learning. Photography by Dino Petrocelli

A well designed and organized supply room can actually save a salon and spa money.

A well-designed and organized supply room can actually save a salon and spa money. Talk to a salon and spa owner, and you will hear, "Supplies are going up," "Our supplies are costing us too much," and "I can't make a profit because of our supply bills." A supply salesman once told me that the most costly supplies that a salon and spa can have are those that do not sell and that sit on the shelves year after year. How much space you give to your supply room, how you take care of your supply inventory, and how you purchase your supplies all have a drastic effect on profits. To get the most from your supply dollar, remember these four rules:

1. Keep an up-to-date inventory on hand at all times.
2. Make and keep a "want list" handy.

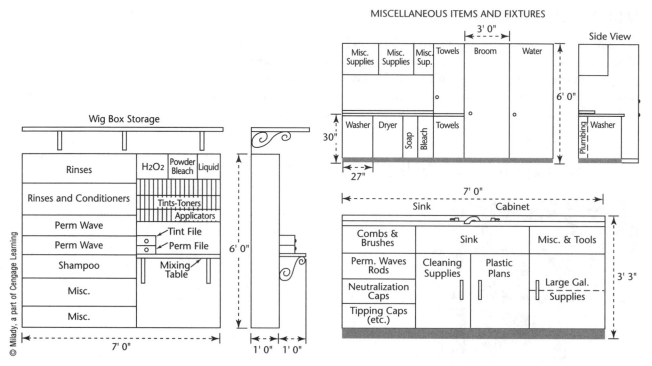

MISCELLANEOUS ITEMS AND FIXTURES

Example of a well organized supple room

3. Place and store merchandise wisely and safely.
4. Take time with your supply representative when placing your order.

Inventory System

An inventory list is a written account of all the products that your salon and spa has on hand. This list should contain everything: items that are used quickly and reordered (shampoo, facial cleaners, massage oils, nail polish, etc.), items that are moderately used and reordered (hair-removal wax, antiseptics, disinfectants, shampoo capes, etc.), items that are seldom used and reordered (styling chair back covers, magazine covers, etc.), and items that are not usually considered back-bar supplies, but are used in the salon and spa (toilet paper, hand soap, coffee cups, etc.). These systems can all be accounted for in a spreadsheet or word-processing program on the computer, or you may prefer a large book that can be ruled for keeping an up-to-date inventory (note the example). Forms and even entire systems for tracking inventory are available from salon and spa educational systems and trade magazines as well as through your distributors.

You can see from the inventory list exactly how much business you are doing in each of the major areas. This also gives you an accurate check of the number of items that were bought and sold. If this figure does not agree with your booked appointments, you know that you have shrinkage somewhere. The inventory sheet is a constant check of the sales (and possibly thefts) in your salon and spa.

With this **inventory system**, you can make accurate purchasing decisions. You can then choose to e-mail, fax, or simply call your order in. As your supplies come in, you can use the inventory system as a check sheet to make sure that you have gotten everything you ordered. If changes were made in the supply order by the distributor, the inventory sheet should be corrected.

inventory system
The process to keep track of objects or materials for the business. Many inventory-control systems rely upon barcodes or RFID tags.

The "Want List"

This list contains the things to be ordered from the inventory sheet and any other things that your technicians might want to order. This list should be posted in the supply room and should be cleared each time that an order is sent in. This "want list" will enable technicians who are not present in the salon and spa at the time that the supply agent arrives to place their order.

Store Merchandise Wisely

In order to take inventory quickly and efficiently, your supplies should be arranged in an orderly fashion. When you are counting the number of tubes of color, you should not have to look in three places to see if there is a tube of a certain color.

When new merchandise comes into the salon and spa, be sure that the old merchandise is brought to the front to be used first; otherwise, the unused supplies will be pushed to the rear and will become old and worthless. Since it is hard to get a technician, front desk associate, or cleaning crew to rotate stock, it is suggested that no supply shelf be more than 1 foot deep. It seems that no one minds moving a bottle or two, but moving six or eight bottles is annoying. Be sure to store cosmetics away from heaters and dryers, as many types spoil in heat. Keep products away from the sink unless they are necessary for shampooing.

The Supply Room/Inventory Design Plan

The supply room can be as complex or as simple as the owner wishes it to be. The larger the salon and spa, the larger the supply room must be. Several ideas for arrangements are given in words and pictures in this chapter. While not all salons and spas can incorporate all of these ideas, they are presented to give you some suggestions on how to improve your supply room. Too often, supply rooms are unorganized, and the cabinets are too large. The result is an untidy supply room with no set pattern to it. This leads to wasted products, overlooked products (causing overpurchasing), and wasted time spent by the technicians looking for supplies.

Floors

Like the floors in the other rooms, the floor in your supply room should be easy to clean and maintain. It should be stain- and soil-resistant.

Cabinets and Sinks

How many? What size? How should they be arranged? These are all questions that management must answer. The more technicians a salon and spa has, the more space is required for a supply room. A double sink is a good idea. A cabinet made of either metal or wood can enclose the sink. If you use a metal cabinet, be sure that it is of the highest quality. Some salon and spa chemicals react with steel, causing it to discolor. The countertop should be molded instead of trimmed. Trimmed cabinets come apart too easily if the Formica comes unglued. If possible, the top of the cabinet should tilt toward the sink for drainage reasons. The cabinet should be at least 3 feet high, 25 inches deep, and from 5 to 7 feet long (note drawing).

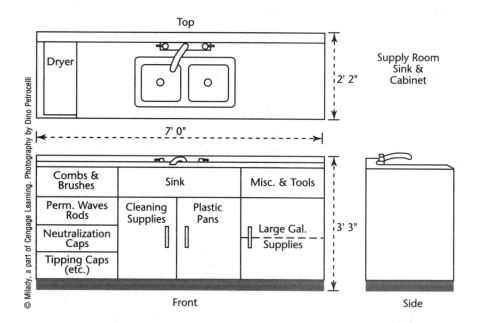

On one side of the sink, there should be drawers, and on the other, shelves. Under the sink is a good place to store plastic buckets and any other containers that are used in cleaning. Cleaning materials should also be kept under the sink; these include:

window cleaner
furniture polish

Inventory Sheet	On Hand January 1, 20 …	Ordered	Received	Total	Used	On Hand February 1, 20…	Ordered	Received	Total	Continued for one year →
Products										
Hair Colors #30	11	12	6	17	9	8	12	12	20	
#32	2	12	12	14	7	7	6	6	13	
#40	5	6	6	11	9	2	12	12	14	
#42	8	12	12	20	12	8	12	10	18	
Perm Waves $00.00 Reg.	24			24	12	12				
Tint	15			15	3	12				
Fine	17	6	6	23	8	15				
Spec.	12			12		12				
Higher priced wave $00.00 Reg.	10	12	12	22	10	12				
Tint	22			22		22				
Fine	5	24	24	29	17	12				
Spec.	7	24	24	31	21	10				

Want List
Shampoo — 4 dozen
Styling Combs — 14
Natural Bristle Brushes — 10
Hot Combs — 2
Hair Spray — 4 dozen
Hair Clips — 4 dozen each
Rollers — Medium and Small — 2 dozen each
Teasing Combs — 8
Styling Razors — 15

sink cleaners
drain cleaners
toilet bowl cleaners
cleaning sponges
cleaning rags, etc.

These cleaning supplies should be placed in a wooden or hard plastic box with handles, as metal will react with some chemicals. Should the sink need repairs, the removal of the cleaning box is quick and simple. Nothing else should go under the sink; this space is not a catchall.

Drawers

On the side of this cabinet should be a row of drawers. The first should contain brushes and combs that are clean, sanitized, and awaiting use. The second drawer should contain permanent wave rods. This drawer should be separated into small, boxlike divisions. Each rod color should be assigned to one of these boxes. This will make rod selection easy and simple. The third drawer should contain processing capes, shampoo capes, comb-out. All plastic coverings should be dried and folded before being placed in the drawer, as a musty odor will result if they are closed in a drawer while still wet.

The fourth drawer is used for processing caps. A heating cap can go in this drawer also. If a manicure heater or manicuring heating gloves are used, they can also go into this drawer. Be sure that electrical cords are placed inside the gloves and cap to prevent a drawer of tangled cords. A manicuring heater can have its cord rolled up and secured with a piece of tape.

Shelves

Your catchall drawer should be on the other side of the sink. This should contain a screwdriver, hammer, measuring tape, and other items for which you need a place. This drawer must be cleaned at least twice a month. It will house many items that should be thrown out at once and, as a result, the drawer will have a tendency to become extremely messy.

Under the catchall drawer, there should be two shelves. These shelves should be large enough to contain cleaning fluids and the boxed, economy-sized supplies for cleaning. Usually, there will be several gallon jugs of cleaning fluid, disinfectant, and wax, and large boxes of comb and brush cleaner, cleaning compounds, and so forth.

Supply Wall

A wall covered with shelves is recommended over cabinets (note drawing). The addition of doors to these shelves will cause them to become disorderly and cluttered. When the supplies are standing out in the open, if they look cluttered, someone will straighten them. Open shelves demand attention and stay neat. These shelves should be about 1 foot wide. They should never be more than 1 foot deep nor less than 9 inches. If the shelves are deeper, staff will not rotate stock because they have to move too many bottles. If the shelves are less than 9 inches deep, a gallon jug will be slightly unstable. The shelves should have a strip of raised trim at the edge to prevent any supplies from falling or rolling off. The shelves should be adjustable in height and anchored well to the wall. Because of the large amount of weight you will be placing on these shelves, they should be well-supported and securely attached to an outside wall when possible.

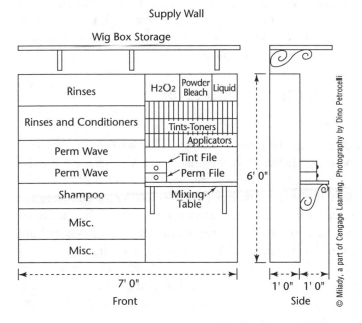

Supply Wall

Shelves should be painted with a good-quality, oil-based paint and washed frequently. The height and length of such a wall will depend on the size of the supply room and the number of employees you have. Refer to the drawing showing such a wall. Note that shelves start at the floor and extend upward 6 feet. If the ceiling in your supply room is over 7 feet tall, a shelf larger than the supply shelves (can be 2 feet wide) could be used for the top shelf and could hold things like wig boxes and other light but bulky items that are not in constant use.

A 2-foot shelf, placed 30 inches from the floor, will serve as a mixing table for tints and permanent waves and will serve as a technician's desk. If a client's tint or permanent wave record is on the computer, a computer terminal may need to be in the supply room. If the table is used for mixing, it should be covered with a good grade of Formica or plastic. The height of this table should allow a chair to be placed under it.

Material Safety Data Sheets (MSDS) Storage

By law, material safety data sheets (MSDS) must be kept on hand and be easily available. Establish a location for these in your supply room in a folder or notebook. Be sure that the sheets are promptly and neatly filed and that everybody knows where they are and how to read them. Since the Occupational Safety and Health Administration (OSHA) regulations governing MSDS use and storage may change, make sure that you remain up-to-date and make any necessary changes in storage as the need arises.

Miscellaneous Items and Fixtures

Washing Machine

Many salons and spas do their own laundry. If a washing machine is purchased, it should be placed on or against a wall that easily provides water and drain connections. Washing machines are generally from 27 to 30 inches wide and about 30 inches deep, including all connections. The back of the machine, where the connections are located, should be closed off and covered to prevent items from being dropped behind them. A good brand of machine that is new or just slightly used is best. An inexpensive washing machine may not hold up to daily washings over a long period of time. Commercial washing machines are excellent for this purpose. Many manufacturers offer service contracts that can save you money in the long run.

Dryer

A dryer is necessary if you have already invested in a washing machine. Dryers also are about 27 inches wide and extend into the room about 30 inches. This depth includes installation and exhaust connections. Be sure that the dryer has a lint filter that can be easily cleaned after each load of wash is dried. This cleaning step will cut down on the cost of operation. If the dryer and washer are on an outside wall, you can vent them directly to the outside without much expense.

Note: Consider purchasing energy-efficient or front-loading washers and dryers, which are more environmentally friendly and cost-effective in the long run.

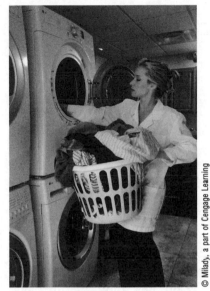

© Milady, a part of Cengage Learning

Energy-efficient or front-loading washers and dryers are environmentally friendly and cost-effective.

Soap and Bleach Cabinet

The cost of soap and bleach are a major factor in doing your own laundry. A commercial bleach and soap (detergent) can be purchased in 100-pound bags and will produce a savings for the salon and spa. The main problem is where to store the products when you have them. A cabinet the same size as your washing machine or dryer will do nicely. Divide the cabinet in half with two bins. These are usually lined with rustproof metal, but if made of wood, they should be covered with plastic to protect them from the soap and bleach. The top of this cabinet, if covered with a good Formica or plastic, makes an excellent place to fold the towels and laundry as they come from the dryer.

Towel/Sheet Storage

Towels are usually kept in the shampoo area. However, you may want an area for overflow. A tall cabinet (6 feet or so) should be located next to the soap and bleach cabinet to house the towels, sheets, and other clean laundry. If this is not convenient, a cabinet above the washer will do just as well. The cabinets should be dustproof if possible and kept cleaned and painted at all times. This cabinet should not contain any other items.

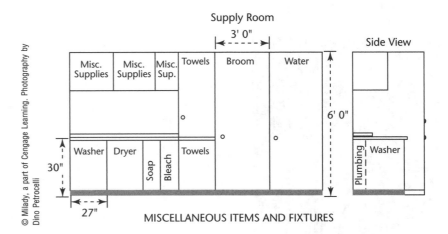

MISCELLANEOUS ITEMS AND FIXTURES

Broom Closet

This closet should be at least 3 feet wide and 3 feet deep. It should contain all cleaning implements, such as brooms, mops, scrub pails, and dustpans. A place for each item should be provided. Hang as many of these items on the wall as you can. This will prevent them from being piled into a corner and creating another mess. This closet should have a tile floor, which should be washed weekly.

Water Heater

Water heaters have changed significantly in the past few years. The standard choices for commercial hot-water tanks or tankless systems are electric and gas, but there are also many businesses that now use solar energy to heat their hot water.

Commercial hot-water heaters without tanks can also be installed outside or inside a building. This can take some stress off contractors and owners who need every square inch for their businesses. However, if you are installing a unit within the business, it can be housed in a closet of its own, or left freestanding in the supply room. If it is freestanding, it should be washed and dusted at least once a week. The size of the water heater will depend upon the size of the salon and spa and the amount of business you intend to do. Most salons and spas have one water heater; however, two smaller heaters connected in series are not uncommon. This can be done so that if either heater should burn out, the other one will take over and work alone until the first is replaced or repaired. If you intend to do your own laundry, be sure that you estimate a higher water and electric bill. Check also with your state board for their requirements.

Standard Equipment

Standard equipment is different from working supplies, as it does not need to be replaced as often. It is different from major appliances and furniture, as it needs to be replaced several times a year, rather than every 10 years or so, as is true of furniture. Bear in mind that some of these items might possibly last one or more years.

Examples:
- Color bowls, color brushes, perm rods, smocks, robes, ceramic coffee cups, wine glasses

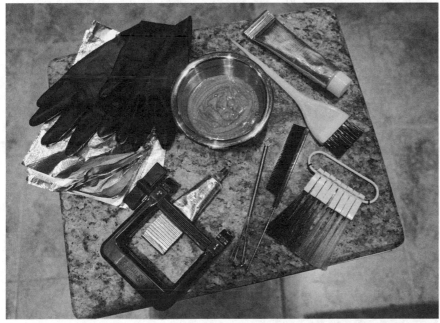

© Milady, a part of Cengage Learning

Standard equipment is different from working supplies.

Cleaning Supplies

Many more items are used in salons and spas that are not mentioned here. These are partial lists of the supplies you might need.

Examples:
- Glass cleaners, wood cleaners, dusters, trash bags

Retail Supplies

Remember that you are stocking two kinds of supplies: items for use in the salon and spa and those to be sold for home use (retail). A good general rule for determining how much retail to keep in stock is to plan on four of each item per technician. Thus, if you have eight technicians, you will need 32 of each item to be sure that you have enough to handle demand. Of course, if you are assertive about retail sales, you may have to stock more, but money will not be wasted as long as the inventory keeps moving out as rapidly as it comes in.

Note: Each separate item is typically referred to as a "SKU" (pronounced "skew," meaning "stock-keeping unit"). If you carry four brands of shampoo, each of which comes in three different formulas according to hair type, you have 12 SKUs of shampoo. Retail should be kept, if possible, in the retail area instead of the supply room. Many retail shelves today are designed to hold the "back stock" in cabinets at the bottom of the shelves. This will free up space and help with shrinkage.

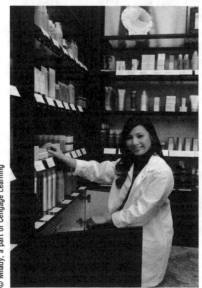

© Millady, a part of Cengage Learning

Retail shelves are designed to hold the "back stock" in cabinets at the bottom of the shelves.

Private Label

Private-label products are available through many distributors. These are good-quality products that carry the salon and spa name on them. You may have to order substantial quantities of these, but the price per item is often lower than for major brands. If your staff *stands behind* the product, *uses it* on their clients, and *promotes it* aggressively, you will benefit from selling private-label products in your salon and spa. Typically, these products are marked up 300 to 500 percent, increasing the profit margin considerably. They also have the advantage of carrying your salon and spa name on the bottle, constantly reminding your client about your salon and spa.

Additional Supplies

In addition to the basic supplies already mentioned, many other items could be housed in your supply room (customize this area for your comfort). A great rule of thumb is "one place for every one item." Also check your state board for their requirements.

Chapter 7 Summary

- A salon and spa has a personality, dependent on original composition, management, operators, supplies and maintenance, and the work it produces. All parts must work well or else the salon and spa will fall into trouble.

- To perform well, management must attend to all parts of the salon and spa, help the staff succeed and participate, and develop management skills.

- Support systems include the bookkeeping system, supply room, supply system, working capital, front desk associate, and maintenance department.

- A well-organized supply room/closet will ultimately save you time and money.

Review Questions

1. What is meant by the "original composition" of the salon and spa? How does the original composition influence the overall success of the salon?

2. Summarize the four things that a salon manager can do to motivate employees.

3. Discuss the importance of one of the support systems listed in this chapter. Include why it is important to a salon and spa business and what you can do to maximize the system's potential.

4. List three good habits that you should develop so that you are able to manage the inventory in your supply room effectively.

5. What are three things that you can do to wisely store your inventory?

Salon and Spa Marketing

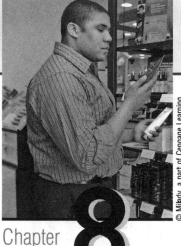

Chapter **8**

When it comes to promoting your salon and spa, marketing is the key to success. It is not so much so about what you spend, but how you spend it. The first thing that you need to consider is the branding of your salon and spa. Marketing your business is multifaceted. This includes your logo, style, slogan, and signage. After you choose your branding, there are a few main categories of marketing. These are **Internet**, **hard copy (print)**, **multimedia**, public relations, and—always our favorite—**word of mouth**. Below is a brief description of these types of marketing and how you can use them in your business.

BASIC BRANDING OF YOUR SALON AND SPA

Branding your salon and spa is a crucial part of your business success development. Simply put, it is how your business is perceived by its customers. Branding is the proprietary visual, emotional, and rational image associated with your salon and spa. Branding is communicating your business's attributes and qualities, and creating a simple but visceral association of those qualities in the minds of your potential customers. For example, if you want a "strong, tough" pickup truck, you probably think of Ford. Toyota, Dodge, and Nissan all build tough pickup trucks, but Ford is the company that has put the most effort into branding their pickup trucks as "tough"—"Built Ford Tough" is their slogan. If you want a quick and inexpensive haircut, you may think of Supercuts or Fantastic Sam's. These examples are large-budget,

Internet
A global system of interconnected computer networks that serve billions of users worldwide.

hard copy
A physical object, permanent reproduction, or copy. Any media suitable for direct use by a person to view displayed or transmitted data.

multimedia
Media and content that use a combination of different content forms, such as a combination of text, audio, still images, animation, video, and interactivity

word of mouth
The passing of information from person to person. What once was literally words from the mouth now includes any type of social communication, such as Facebook, e-mail, text messaging, and telephone.

branding
A sign, name, or symbol used to identify a business, service, or specific product.

logo
A graphic mark or emblem to aid and promote instant public recognition. Logos are either purely graphic (symbols/icons) or composed of the name of the organization.

slogan
A memorable motto or phrase used as a repetitive expression of an idea or purpose for the business.

widespread branding efforts, but smaller businesses brand their images as well. The purpose of having people remember the brand name and have positive associations with that brand is to make their selection easier and enhance the value and satisfaction they get. You should consider what type of image you want for your salon and spa, and what type of clientele you wish to attract. Make sure that these concepts work together, not against each other.

- Create a compelling name for your salon and spa.
- Create a **logo** and "style guide" for your salon and spa. Having a good-quality logo and style guide for your salon and spa is an important element of branding your salon and spa's image in the public mind. Do you have a quality logo that represents the level of professionalism offered by your salon and spa? Does your color scheme invoke the correct type of visceral response in potential customers' minds, or is it a rainbow of randomness?
- Create a **slogan** (or series of slogans) that defines the qualities your business has that may set it apart from the competition. Even if you do not publically market or use a slogan, it is a good idea for you to develop one for internal use and focus. This might be part of a "mission statement." What are the key attributes of your business that set it apart from other similar businesses?
- Install attractive signage on your building and around your business location. Try to put yourself in a third party's perspective and drive by or walk by your location. Does your business stand out, or does it blend into the surroundings? Do you have prominent, clear signage that identifies your core business as a salon and spa? If possible, consider posting additional permanent or temporary signage near your location to catch more eyes.

USING THE INTERNET/WEB

The latest U.S. census figures show that over 60 percent of U.S. households are now connected to the Web, and that percentage is projected to rise over the coming years. The percentage is even higher for younger households and households with over $50,000 in annual income. An increasing number of consumers are using the Internet to find products and services, and to locate businesses in their area. In order to keep up with the fast pace and remain competitive, creating and promoting a Web site for your salon and spa should be a key element of your business marketing strategy. Web sites, blogs, podcasts, banners, pop-up ads, e-mail, and chat rooms are all **cyber platforms** that allow promotional content to be available 24/7. Creating a Web site involves three basic steps.

Getting the Web Site Built

A Web site is nothing more than a bunch of files, both graphic and text, that are woven together around a common theme. The cost for developing the site can be anywhere from $299 to $2,000 (and up), depending on size and functions. For most basic small-business sites, the cost will run between $500 and $1,000. This cost is a one-time investment for a tool you own and can continue to use for communication and marketing.

You may also consider the do-it-yourself option. Today, there are many tools online that make creating your own Web site fairly simple. Creating pages for the Web takes a little practice, but once you get the hang of it, it is a lot of fun. There are several free online tutorials illustrating a step-by-step guide that will show you how to create it yourself.

Hosting

Once the site is built, it must be hosted on a public server so the general public can access it through Internet providers. **Hosting** costs vary. They can run anywhere from $4 to $50 per month, based on the Web site functionality and the hosting provider. Service varies widely as well. The ideal host will offer several services bundled together for one affordable price. The space provided for your site on the server should have ample room for high traffic (bandwidth). When a site does not have enough bandwidth, the Web visitor finds the site slow-loading and difficult to access. The hosting package should have at least one e-mail address that can be accessed through the Web. The hosting package should have a reliable track record of maintaining high dependability. When your server goes down, your Web site and associated e-mail are unavailable.

Domain Name

A **domain name** is the Web address where users find your Web site (www.yourcompany.com). Domain names are unique and cannot be duplicated. The cost for registering a unique domain name can vary greatly from zero cost (with a time restriction) up to $35 per year.

cyber platform
An Internet environment used as platforms for ad delivery.

Web hosting
A hosting service that allows the salon and spa site to be accessible via the World Wide Web.

domain name
An identification label that defines a realm of administrative autonomy, authority, or control on the Internet.

search-engine optimization
The process of improving the visibility of a Web site in search engines.

e-mail marketing
The use of e-mail as a means of communicating commercial or fund-raising messages to bring customers to the business and generate sales.

Online Networking Sites

Search-Engine Optimization

Search-engine optimization improves your Web site's position in all the major search engines, such as Google, Yahoo, MSN, AOL, InfoSeek, AltaVista, AskJeeves, and others. Organic search-engine optimization comprises all the tricks of savvy Web design that get you "free exposure" through the regular results of the search engines.

E-mail Marketing

E-mail addresses collected on the site or in your establishment are stored in your e-mail database; you can then develop custom e-mail promotions to send out to all of your customers. Best of all, **e-mail marketing** campaigns are free, no matter how many you send—no postage required.

Social Networking Sites

Facebook, MySpace, Bebo, Twitter, and so forth are all forms of marketing on "social networks." These all can be a fairly simple and hands on way to promote your business. Of course, we all like things

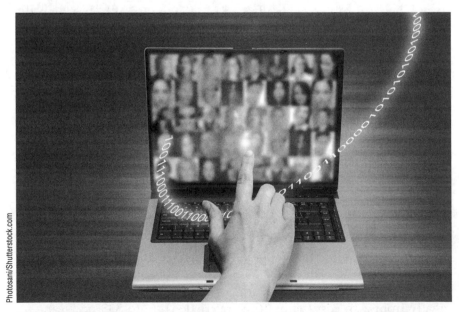

Photosani/Shutterstock.com

Social-networking Web sites can be very effective in cost and strategy.

to be free, but with the right message, many businesses—small businesses especially—will find the marketing abilities of these **social-networking Web sites** to be very effective in cost and strategy.

PRINT MARKETING FOR YOUR SALON AND SPA

Direct Mail

Because most of a salon and spa's clients usually come from an area surrounding the salon and spa—a 5-mile radius is typically where 90 percent of most salon and spa clients live or work—direct mail makes a lot of sense. Delivering to local homes/businesses can be inexpensive. Also, direct mail is the best way both to entice first-time visitors to return to your salon and spa and to keep your present clients informed and interested in your services, products, and promotions. A discount on first-time services may be offered. One idea is to find other local businesses that may share a similar client base and do a cross-promotion mailing. For example, if you have a standard hair salon, consider partnering with a day spa, tanning spa, or massage therapist. Also consider sending out mail to potential new clients who are new to the area.

Yellow Pages

Traditional yellow-page marketing should be a part of your basic marketing plan, but many salons and spas are turning away from expensive yellow-page ads and focusing on marketing that provides a higher return on investment (ROI). Things to consider when comparing your yellow-page ad with your competition's ad: Are you wasting space? Are you conveying your key slogan or key quality of your salon and spa that sets you apart from the competition?

Flyers, Posters

A professional flyer/poster is an inexpensive and highly effective way to grab attention and to promote your business, products, services, and events. They are also a wonderful—not to mention effective—marketing tool for new business start-ups as well as established businesses with budgetary constraints.

social networking site
An online platform or site that focuses on building and reflecting social relations among people who share interests and/or activities.

Newspaper Ads

Although the popularity of the tangible newspapers has faded, many people are now choosing to read them online. Regardless of their form, they are still an option for salons and spas to consider for marketing their services. Consider smaller neighborhood papers, as well as larger city (or even national) newspapers. If your business is located in a small town, marketing in the local community paper makes sense; that way, you can attract the locals who would most likely frequent your store. If your business or service is specific to a particular section of the newspaper, run your ad in that area of the paper.

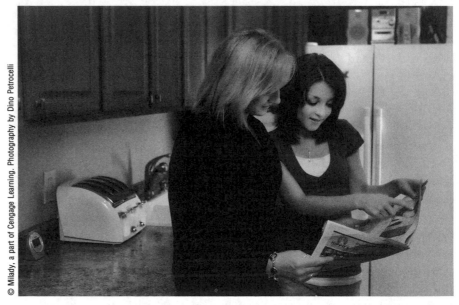

© Milady, a part of Cengage Learning. Photography by Dino Petrocelli

You may want to consider smaller neighborhood papers in addition to larger ones.

RADIO OR TELEVISION MARKETING

Radio and television marketing can be expensive, and you may find it inappropriate for single-location salons or spas, but if you have several locations within a region, consider regional radio or television ads. Be sure to track referrals from radio or television so you can analyze the ROI and compare to your other marketing mediums. Contact your local sales managers at television and radio stations in your area and arrange to have a salesperson visit you. However, with that said, you may find at times that they have "overstock," which means that they may be able to trade services for marketing. You also may be able to provide services for the local anchors in exchange for marketing.

PUBLIC RELATIONS

Business Lunches

Business lunches or morning breakfasts of such groups as the Chamber of Commerce, the Lions Club, Junior League, and Rotary are good avenues to male clients. The salon and spa can coordinate hairstyles. A lecture on hair and nail care or spa services is good marketing. Be sure to have a number of before-and-after pictures available for viewing.

Style Shows and Demonstrations

Style shows and demonstrations are a great form of marketing for a salon and spa because you have the attention of an interested, captive audience. The people to whom you are demonstrating are interested in what you have to say and will listen. Each hairstyle you create during a demonstration should be explained, and the care of it should be discussed. Related subjects, such as coloring, bleaching, or updos, can all be introduced while you are working on the model.

Marketing through Conventions and Educational Seminars

Conventions and seminars are a real learning experience. When a technician returns, he or she will have some new ideas, some new styles, and some new ambitions. The salon and spa should capitalize on this. When the technician or manager returns, an ad should be run to inform clients. A perfect place to inform clients of this type of information would be on Facebook, MySpace, Bebo, or Twitter.

Example:
"The Hair First salon's team has returned from New York, where they have been attending a hairstyling seminar. They have brought

back with them many new hairstyles suited to the new fall clothing." You can add photos to share the experience visually and to create excitement.

The added business from such an ad sometimes pays for the trip. The main thing to remember is that if you are going to do something, let someone know about.

Clubs and Organizations

When you are offered a chance to join a club or organization, do so. You may not want to be an officer of the organization, but the exposure to other members will stimulate business. If employees have a chance to join an organization, encourage them to do so. In fact, if you have to pay their dues, do so. Each time you or a member of your salon and spa staff is seen socially, the topic of the salon and spa is bound to come up. In each case, it is a chance to market your salon and spa. The more your salon and spa personnel become involved with the community, the larger your salon and spa profits will be.

Always carry plenty of business cards. Hand them out to everybody you meet, and be proud of what you do. "Talk up" your salon and spa and its services at every opportunity; pride and excitement are contagious.

Welcome Wagons and Newcomers' Clubs

Some communities have organizations such as the Welcome Wagon and Newcomers' Club. These organizations call upon new community members and welcome them to the area. They give the newcomer gift items and list the merchants who wish to say hello. A free gift such as a pen (with your salon and spa name on it) will give you a lot of marketing. Some salons and spas give newcomers special rates on services for their first visit. All these things market the salon and spa and generate word-of-mouth marketing.

Charity/Donations

Charitable giving for small businesses is truly a valuable contribution to our quality of life. Many small businesses are generous and wish to donate to worthy causes. Make sure you understand the basics of small-company charitable giving. You may choose to offer gift cards as donations in order to get new clients into the salon and spa. People tend to take advantage of things that are free, or where the proceeds go to a charity the client supports. They may not have had knowledge of your salon and spa until they receive a gift certificate from a donation, or stop by the salon and spa to participate in the charitable event.

Public-service marketing conveys socially relevant messages about important matters and social-welfare causes. These topics can range from cancer, to global warming, to child abuse, to illiteracy, to poverty. David Ogilvy once said, "Marketing justifies its existence when used in the public interest—it is much too powerful a tool to use solely for commercial purposes."

Note: Today, television and radio stations are granted a fixed number of public-service marketings aired by the channel.

■ SALON AND SPA ADVERTISEMENTS

Salon and Spa Conversation—A Form of Marketing

If technicians are not talking to one another in the salon and spa, you are missing one of the best forms of marketing. The talking should not be going on all the time, nor should it distract from the client, but it is a very good form of marketing. During the course of the day, you might ask a nearby technician, "Jan, how do you like your new hair color?" This is like a spot-marketing notice in the store. Immediately, all eyes in the salon and spa will turn to Jan. As Jan says she likes it, all the operators and clients will automatically start talking about hair color. This type of marketing is quite effective and is a good way to break up a day's work. If it is done too often, however, it will lose its effectiveness.

There are several ways you can promote good **public relations** in a salon and spa. Here are three ways:

1. *The manager speaks to each customer entering the salon and spa.* If the manager does not know the person's name, he or she can wait until the person is seated at a technician's chair and take the name from the appointment schedule. Everyone likes to be noticed. The greatest recognition is the one in which you mention a person's name. "Hello, Mrs. Jones. It sure is a nice day today." This type of greeting will keep customers in the salon and spa year after year.

2. *Technician–client relations must be on a personal level.* This can be as simple as taking a client's coat, brushing his or her suit off after a hair shaping, or saying "happy birthday." To do this well, each technician should have a file on each of his or her steady customers. When something important happens, it should be noted and

public relations
The maintenance and/or enhancement of a business's or organization's public image and reputation.

mentioned to the client the next time he or she comes into the salon and spa. This information can be easily stored in a notes section in the salon and spa computer. If not computerized, you may choose to keep this information on the client cards.

3. *Take bad public relations out of complaints.* One of the most difficult things to handle in the salon and spa is the complaint. The client is usually upset, and the more he or she talks about his or her trouble, the more emotional he or she becomes. The first thing to do is to talk softly and find out what the problem is. Next, admit nothing until you have spoken to your technician, but try to find out what the client wants to have done. In the case of unsatisfactory work, try to have him or her return to the salon and spa to have the problem corrected. If an adjustment is in order, make it as quickly and quietly as possible. The client may not like what he or she has experienced, but if the situation is handled carefully, he or she will not damage your salon and spa reputation with all of his or her neighbors.

Sales and Specials

Sales and specials have been used for years, and their attraction has to do with special lower prices or gifts. These sales promotions are still drawing people into salons and spas. Salons and spas use this form of marketing to do two things: stimulate sales and remove old merchandise from the shelves. Holding too many sales is not good for a salon and spa, as the salon and spa can get the reputation of being a cut-rate operation.

The best time for a sale is when business is at a low during the year; during the peak season, it could be a disaster. Promotions should follow a specific cycle. Four weeks is a good length for a promotion. The expiration date encourages people to try it before it runs out.

WORD-OF-MOUTH MARKETING

Word-of-mouth marketing is the most effective marketing as well as the least expensive. What makes for good word-of-mouth marketing? First, you must stimulate your clients to talk about your salon and spa in a favorable way. This is achieved by your conversations with them when they are in your salon and spa. Make sure to give your client all your time. When the client first sits down in your chair, inquire about what he or she wants out of the service. Ask the client about previous experiences and what he or she liked or disliked about those experiences. If the client wishes to talk, make sure you do your best to remain positive. Be sure he or she is happy with your services. Second, be sure that the client always looks his or her best when he or she leaves your salon and spa.

Here are four hints to keep in mind when you are seeking this type of marketing:

1. Always keep your clients looking their best.
2. When working on a client, give him or her your complete attention. Avoid talking to other operators or clients too often.
3. Technicians should give clients helpful hints on how to maintain a hairstyle. This should be some simple, workable advice that the client can pass on to his or her friends.
4. Never underestimate simply asking the client for a referral.

ABOVE ALL—RECORD-KEEPING

Be sure to keep a record of all the ads that you have run. You can easily store them on your computer, CDs, flash drives, or hard copies—whatever you are comfortable with. As time goes by, you will find this extremely helpful. Not only will you not have to reinvent the wheel, but it is a great insight to your business's growth. This will also allow you to understand whether the marketing worked. Make the following notations:

1. How many calls came in from the ad
2. How many appointments were booked
3. What services were rendered and whether they prebooked any further services.
4. What and how many retail products were purchased
5. A record of new customers who responded
6. The dollar amount spent and earned on the promotion

Be sure to keep a scrapbook or other notes on the marketing done by other businesses in your area. It can provide a few ideas for future ads of your own. Remember, the more detailed your record-keeping, the more successful your future marketing will be.

Note: Several other marketing plans are used by salons and spas throughout the country. Keep in mind that the main principle behind marketing is to attract clients to you so they will buy what you are selling!

Chapter 8 Summary

- The first thing that you need to consider is the branding of your salon and spa.

- Creating and promoting a Web site for your salon and spa should be a key element of your business marketing strategy if you want to be competitive now and in coming years.

- The five main forms of marketing include Web, hard copy, radio/television, public relations, and in-salon and spa marketing.

- Word-of-mouth marketing is the most effective and cheapest type of marketing.

- The more detailed your record-keeping, the more successful your future marketing will be.

Review Questions

1. In what ways can you use a slogan? What should you consider when writing it?

2. List three Internet resources for marketing and how you would use each of them specifically.

3. List at least two benefits of using direct-mail marketing.

4. What are three things that technicians can do to increase word-of-mouth marketing?

5. Discuss at least three important pieces of information regarding your marketing that need to be recorded and why that information is important to you.

Merchandising in Your Salon and Spa

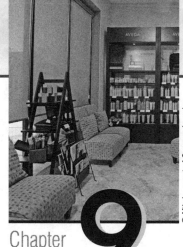

Chapter **9**

"**H**ow are sales?" "How is business?" These are common questions that are asked when salon and spa owners get together. The answers to these questions are as confusing as the questions themselves. One manager might think of business in terms of customer service, while another may consider the overall operation of the salon and spa. From these questions and answers, we find that many owners and managers may not comprehend the full meaning of the salon and spa business.

Let us start by defining a few terms in this chapter:

Merchandising in the salon and spa is the total of activities related to selling all goods, services, and retail items that one might find in a salon and spa.

Gross sales are the total amount of money taken in by the salon and spa during the year.

Net profit is the difference between the cost of goods and services and their selling price. Labor would be part of the cost of a shampoo/ style service as well as the shampoo and hair spray.

Real profit is a term used to describe the amount of money left after all bills have been paid.

MAIN STEPS IN MERCHANDISING

All it takes is a trip to the local mall. There are hundreds and hundreds of retail merchandise displays designed to entice and cajole the consumer into buying. Merchandising, or how retail products are arranged

merchandising
The methods, practices, and operations used to promote and sustain certain products and/or services within the business.

gross sales
The total amount of money taken in by the salon and spa during the year; overall sales, before deducting operating expenses, cost of goods sold, payment of taxes, or any other expenses.

net profit
The difference between the cost of goods and services and their selling price. Labor, as well as the shampoo and hair spray, would be part of the cost of a shampoo/style service.

109

real profit
The amount of money left after all bills have been paid.

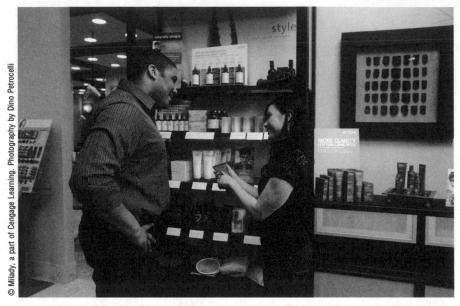

Set the stage for a positive selling environment.

and displayed on your shelves, sets the stage for a positive selling environment. With this in mind, let us explore how to merchandise in a salon and spa. This chapter centers around three main processes and how to use them. If these steps are followed, the salon and spa will prosper and grow.

1. Getting customers into the salon and spa.
2. Giving customers what they want.
3. Selling/servicing customers needs

Getting Customers into the Salon and Spa

The first thing you want to consider is, "What makes a customer come into a salon and spa?" Some of the frequently heard answers to this question are the location, the appearance, and the marketing—that is, the Web site, Internet, print work, and good recommendations. All of these and many more are applicable to all salon and spa owners. In addition, a salon and spa must launch and maintain an active program to get customers into the salon and spa and retain them as customers. When you are talking about spending money in business, you do not want to gamble. You invest it wisely. Presented here are a few items that work. However, keep your eyes and mind open for new ideas that appear to fit your business.

Planning

First make a plan, and then follow it. In setting up the plan, consider the following questions.

1. What type of customers are you looking for?
2. What type of customer currently comes into your salon and spa?
3. What types of businesses are near your salon and spa? What is their traffic pattern?
4. Can you tie in with their marketing program for the benefit of your salon and spa?
5. Do you wish to change the type of customers you already have, or do you just wish to add a few more?
6. Should you consider changing your location? (If your goal is young, fashion-forward clientele, you would not want to be in a retirement community.)

Take the time; answer all these questions. Remember, a well-laid-out plan will enable you to be proactive, not reactive.

Example:

The name of our salon and spa is Urban Chic Salon and Spa, located in the Hillcrest area of San Diego. Its know to be a high pedestrian traffic area, The average customers are young professionals with two years of college, in their late twenties to early forties, who live and work in the area and are looking to be trendsetters This area serves a diverse but youthful clientele.

The objective is to increase the number of customers while keeping the present ones.

Our salon and spa is close to the major pedestrian traffic centers in the shopping area. Remember, the first step is all about location, location, location. Next, we may want to contact the shops and boutiques next to us and see what they are doing in terms of promotion. Each month, merchants have a theme to draw customers. Monthly specials work for some types of salons and spas, but not all. Higher-end salons and spas may gain clientele in part by their sense of exclusivity. Your salon and spa does not need to have a special every month, but it is important to have different ideas to reference. Let the merchants who do a lot of marketing set the theme of the promotions and sales. If the dress boutique has a pre-spring sale, and it is located next door to our salon and spa, we will take advantage of it by decorating our window to read "Swing into Spring with a New Hairstyle." Use colors that will blend—but will not be overpowered by—our neighbor's display.

Since this is a shopping center (with a regular group of customers), chances are that people are used to shopping in the same stores. Our window display will attract some, yet others may not see it, so reinforcement is needed. Since this is a dress sale, have the clerks in the dress store come in for a new spring hairdo. When Mrs. Gonzales goes in to purchase a new dress, she sees store clerk Hailee's hair and comments about it. This is good for two reasons: first, Hailee is flattered, and second, the customer is told where Hailee got her new hairstyle. The cost of this type of marketing is very low, and the results pay off.

Salon and Spa Appearance

The overall appearance of a salon and spa is a real asset to your business. Attractive windows and doors have already been discussed, but they are so important to business that they are worth mentioning again. Clean windows with attractive displays, changed every 3 weeks, are real business-builders.

Be sure that the waiting retail area is well-lit and open, so a passerby can see into the salon and spa at night. The cost is low, and benefits—both for marketing and protection—are large.

New Client Promotions

Some salons and spas offer discounts to attract new clients. One way you may market your salon and spa is by offering discount prices through services. The discount is usually offered to the new clients on their first visit to the salon and spa. As an alternative to a discount, you can offer a free retail gift with the first hair or spa service, and you will have introduced one of your high-profit retail items to a potential buyer.

Meetings and Training Seminars

It is a good idea to hold staff meetings at least once a month. The owner/manager may lead the meeting. Having a guest stylist or teacher speak creates excitement. These meetings can last from about 30 minutes to a couple of hours, and attendance should be mandatory for all staff members. Be sure these meetings are well-planned, interesting, and interactive.

Some of the topics that may be discussed during these meetings are human relations, communication, salesmanship, new service techniques, new products, and the service and retail sales results.

Since you have made some effort to get clients into the salon and spa, help your technicians with ideas to retain them. Manufacturers, distributors, and salon and spa educators offer this instruction; seek them out and let them help you. One important thing to remember is that while you might own the salon and spa, the technicians *are* the business.

Electronic Media

Many fine training programs are offered in various **electronic media** from salon and spa education companies, spanning every subject, from technical trainings to client-service training. The training aids can stimulate lively discussions. You can also construct your own program using the materials mentioned.

School Demonstrations

Demonstrations in schools are always welcomed and represent a source of future staff and customers. The one thing you must know is the audience to whom you are going to present education and what their ages are. Keep in mind that today's youth are well-versed on up-and-coming fashions, and in many cases are the trendsetters themselves, so your education presentations need to be relevant to your audience.

Using the Web

The Internet is a source of marketing if used properly. For many, the first introduction to your salon and spa will be your Web site. This is one of the most powerful and cost-effective direct-marketing tools you will develop, and one that will virtually market itself. The more places to which you can link yourself, the more visibility your Web site will receive. By having your information connected to multiple places online, it is more likely that your information will pop up in search engines, yellow pages, online networking, and so forth. It is important to remember that you want your information to be relevant to the places to which it is connected. The Web has its own language, which often seems like a great deal of technology; however, do not feel overwhelmed. There are Web host providers and/or information technology consultants that can be a great resource in helping you to maximize your visibility.

Word of Mouth

Nothing but good can come to a salon and spa that has its clients working for it. **Word of mouth** is the best type of marketing and always will be. Doctors, dentists, and attorneys have relied on this type of marketing for years. If your salon and spa has a customer who has sent you a client, be sure to acknowledge him or her—this can be anything from a thank-you note or a small gift to a complete rewards program. A new

electronic media
Media that use electronic or electromechanical energy for the end user to access the content.

word of mouth
The passing of information from person to person. What once was literally words from the mouth now includes any type of social communication, such as Facebook, e-mail, text messaging, and telephone.

and steady client can mean hundreds of dollars per year to a salon and spa, and this type of lead deserves a "thank you."

In thanking a person, be sure to mention the name of the new customer:

> "Mrs. Gonzales, I want to thank you for recommending our salon and spa to Mrs. Roberts." You might even add, "Please accept this gift as a token of our appreciation."

These techniques for getting the customer into the salon and spa have, no doubt, brought other ideas to your mind. At this point, write them down in your notebook and form a plan of action.

"Bring-a-friend" promotions often produce excellent results. Offer a free discount or free products to new clients, and do not forget to present your clients who referred them.

Note: The happier your present clients are with your service, the better this promotion works.

Giving Customers What They Want

When clients come into the salon and spa, they are looking for two things—service and satisfaction. Upon arrival, greet the person immediately, whether it is his or her first visit or hundredth visit. Should the person have to wait, offer a magazine or a cup of coffee to help pass the time.

When the person is placed in the styling chair/table/room, be sure to listen to what the client wants. The first visit should be the time for the client to get to know the salon and spa and the technicians. The first and main objective of this visit is to gain the person's confidence and to get to know one another.

Ask the Right Questions

Ask questions that enhance the customer's experience. Keep in mind that customers purchase two things: good feelings and solutions. With a few simple questions, you can easily gather this information.

1. Confirm that you will be asking a few brief questions to better service the customer today.
2. Establish a time line: "When was the last time you received a haircut (wax/facial etc.)?" This will allow the customer's mind to focus and will give you valuable information about his or her patterns.
3. "What did you like about your last haircut (hair color, manicure, etc.)?" This will give you valuable information about what works currently for the client.

4. "What do you not like about your haircut (hair color, manicure, etc.)?" This will tell you what needs to be changed.

5. "What would you like to change today about your haircut (hair color, manicure, etc.)?" This will tell you what the client sees as his or her needs and what the client wants to change.

6. "What are your currently using for products?" This will allow you to understand what products the client is currently using, and how to better serve his or her product needs.

7. "How is it working for you?"

Once a client is in for a service, you need to understand what he or she wants and needs. From this short conversation, the smart stylist has learned several important things about this customer. They should be written on the client's record card and used for sales later.

Ask the Client to Return

The most important thing is that the technician invites the client back to the salon and spa. A sample exchange follows:

Technician: "I'd like to see you back in about four weeks to maintain your next haircut. Would four or five weeks be better for you?"

CLIENT: "five weeks."

Technician: "Which is better, the beginning or the end of the week?"

Client: "Beginning."

Technician: "Would Tuesday or Wednesday work for you?"

Client: "Wednesday."

Technician: "Which is better, morning or afternoon?"

Client: "Morning."

Technician: "I have a 10:00 a.m., will that work?

Client: "Yes."

Technician: "Great, we will see you Wednesday, August 4, at 10:00 a.m. Let me get you a reminder card."

If the client says he or she does not want to rebook:

Technician: "Well, Mrs. Gonzales, I understand what you are saying. However, I want to make sure that there is time available for you to see Marissa. So why don't we go ahead and book the appointment. I will call you the day before to remind you and we will see how that works for you."

If the client still prefers to call in, the technician/front desk associate should give the technician's card to the client. If no response is forthcoming in a month, be sure the client receives a follow-up call or e-mail. This is a nice way to say, "We enjoy your business."

Selling/Servicing Customers' Needs

Ask yourself this question: When you say *retail*, what comes to mind? You may think of such things as *selling, too expensive, not my job, pushy, pressure*; the owner is the only one who makes the money. How many of you have ever experienced being "sold"? Now, ask another question: How many of you have ever experienced being *served*? Being served means being so completely taken care of that you buy whatever the technician recommends. When you are *served*, not *sold*, you feel welcomed, great, happy, willing to buy, and important. Can you tell that true retailing is about serving the client, not selling to the client? It is about education and helping clients get what *they* want, not what *you* want. When you serve the client, it is fun, the client loves it, and the client buys the products he or she needs to keep him or her looking and feeling beautiful.

This type of selling/servicing will greatly increase salon and spa profits. You may choose to give a small commission on each item to the technician or front desk associate. One idea you may consider is paying this with a separate check, at a separate time from regular paychecks. This will focus more attention on the monies earned from retail product sales. Also, if you keep a chart of retail performance, noting each technician's performance over time and his or her performance compared with others for the month will be an excellent motivational tool. Sales and selling take very little extra effort, and the profits will startle you.

A good front desk associate can also increase the gross income of a salon and spa with additional services or product. When a client is calling in or rebooking his or her appointments, a front desk associate should always ask if the client wants an additional service or products.

HOW TO PURCHASE, MARKET, AND SELL RETAIL ITEMS

Generally speaking, all purchasing should be done by one person. The items purchased should fall into two classes: usable items (back stock) and retail items (items for resale). Ordering is governed by the inventory sheet. Amounts of such items should fall into a pattern reflecting the traffic flow of the salon and spa. Care should be taken to supply the salon and spa with an adequate stock. Your distributor can give you many statistics to support you in your initial purchases. It is not in their best interest to overstock you, as they should plan on a long-term relationship with you and your business.

Selecting Retail Lines

The lines you choose will have a lot to do with your success in retail sales. Here are some important points to keep in mind when selecting lines:

1. Do not buy into too many product lines. Be cautious not to over-whelm the clients and service technicians with too many options. It is also important for the products you sell to be in sync with your salon and spa's philosophy.
2. Be sure the product lines are popular with your staff, as technicians usually sell most effectively when they understand and like a product.
3. Be sure the product lines are sold exclusively to salons and spas. Any diversion (sales to mass marketers) will undermine your sales and your credibility. If you do find one of your lines being sold in local mass markets, contact the distributor and manufacturer. If you do not get satisfaction, drop that line.
4. You are buying into a distributor, not just a product line. Go with the distributor who offers you the most promotional help with such offers as shrink wraps, promotions, special deals, education, and so forth. Build a relationship with this distributor instead of wasting your time saving nickels and dimes on a few products.

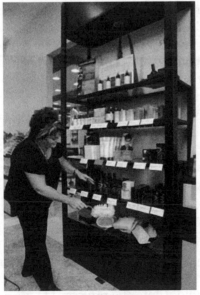

© Milady, a part of Cengage Learning. Photography by Dino Petrocelli

Choosing which retail lines to carry is an important decision.

Retail Items

Choosing which retail items to sell is by far the most important decision. Before entering this field, ask yourself the following questions:

1. Who are my customers?
2. What will their purchasing needs be?
3. Are these products only sold in professional salons and spas?
4. What educational support system will the distributor offer?

In most cases, the product will be priced at twice the purchase price. This amounts to a 50 percent markup because 50 percent of the product's retail price is markup. While this price may vary, the 50 percent markup is a good rule of thumb for specialty stores such as salons and spas, where professional recommendations are very important and where merchandising does not rely on the high turnover of mass marketing. If the technician and front desk associate are going to do the selling/servicing, it is a good idea to reward them financially as stated above. The customers in most areas require different things at different times. One item or a group of related items should be featured each month or, at the very least, every couple months.

■ THE YEARLY PROMOTION

This is where being proactive versus reactive will come in handy. Once you have established your customers' needs, you are now ready to set up yearly promotion programs. You must adapt it to your own area and clientele, and remember that it takes time to build up a demand for new types of merchandise. Do not suddenly go into selling clothing or jewelry in a big way. You need to make a long-term commitment, and start small, to see if it will work without risking too much of your capital.

It is a good idea to use a basic, consistent template each year. This can easily be done in numerous ways. It is highly suggested that once you have created your promotions, you keep them on a CD or flash drive. You may also create monthly bins for promotional tangible items, such as decorations, posters, flyers, and so forth.

Note: The key to making any rewards program work is to make it a positive situation for both the employee and the salon and spa owner. Money is a strong motivator, but it is not the only motivator; find out exactly what inspires your staff and build it into the program. Is it time off, paid education, or a monetary bonus at the end of the week, month, or year? Experience has taught that the more specific a promotion is, the easier it is to gauge the success of it, and so you will know whether it is worth doing again.

January: New Year, New You

Enter to win a complimentary makeover by our entire staff.

The Plan

Have clients and potential customers submit photos and letters explaining what they would like to change about their appearance and why they want to have a makeover. Select numerous candidates to undergo the transformation. Make sure you have a photographer on hand to capture the moments. Tie in your makeover contest with a local talk show and add it on your Web site; you could even make posters out of before and after shoots to place in and around your salon and spa.

Reward (all staff)

Bragging rights! Plus, Who ever participates in the make over will have a featured spot on your Web site, if you choose to display the work on your walls, their name can be placed on the photo for all your consumers to see. You could also have them be a participant on the local talk shows

Staff Promotions: You should constantly promote your staff to boost morale, reward hard workers, and call clients' attention to your employees' abilities. Staff promotions could include incentives, choosing a "Stylist of the Month," displaying the staff's educational certificates, and featuring a different staff member in each newsletter.

■ ■ ■

February: Lip Service

Any client who tries one of our lip colors is invited to be in the contest.

The Plan

After trying on a lip color, each client kisses a little card to make a lip imprint and writes his or her name and address on the other side of the card. At the end of the month, your staff votes for the "cutest lips." The winner receives a makeup kit.

The Reward (all staff)

Each guest is worth 1 point. Each staff member needs to get at least 10 guests per week to participate and to purchase a makeup item. This could earn your business additional monies in retail sales. A staff member needs 30 points to receive a complimentary travel-sized product.

■ ■ ■

March: Shamrock Shopping

Hang shamrocks throughout the retail area. Each client chooses a shamrock, which on the back reveals a prize ranging from a percentage off a retail product to a complimentary salon and spa service.

The Plan

Buy shamrocks at the local party store. For prizes, include services with newer technicians who need clients, or give away products you are trying to move. This promotion is typically done during a slow time.

The Reward (all staff)

Each guest is worth 1 point. For every 10 guests who purchase two or more products each, the staff member receives a predetermined dollar amount for an approved educational class.

■ ■ ■

April: Poker Night

For 1 month, a deck of cards and luck determine the discount percentage on a purchase of three or more retail products.

The Plan

When a client purchases three or more products at once, he or she picks a card from a standard deck of playing cards. If it is a number card, the client receives 10 percent off the purchase; a face card earns 15 percent off; and an ace means 20 percent off. A poster in the front desk area explains the promotion.

The Reward (all staff)

Each guest is worth 1 point. Each staff member needs to get at least 10 guests per week to participate and to purchase a makeup item. Each guest will earn the staff member 1 point. This will earn you additional monies in retail sales. A staff member needs 30 points to receive a complimentary travel-sized product.

■ ■ ■

May: Mother's Day Makeovers

The salon and spa partners with a local radio station to do a Mother's Day promotion. The salon and spa gives away four makeovers, manicures, and one grand-prize package of a makeover, manicure, pedicure, and massage. The mothers are nominated by write-in stories from their children or loved ones about why they deserve the prize.

The Plan

All of the marketing is done through a radio station a couple weeks before the promotion. Do a live interview discussing the contest—how to submit entries to the radio station, and how a group from the station will pick the winners. The week of Mother's Day, a winner is announced every day on the radio.

The Reward (all staff)

Sure to be a staff favorite each year. The reward is simply a feel good. The stories that will be sent in will amaze you, it's hard not to get wrapped up in outpourings or love between a mother and child.

■ ■ ■

June: Summer Camp for Dad

The salon and spa opens on Father's Day to allow fathers a day of fun and relaxation.

The Plan

The spa partners with a local golf course to provide a package including golf and a salon and spa day.

The Reward (all staff)

For every two guests the staff member books for the summer camp promotion, the staff member will receive a pair of movie tickets.

■ ■ ■

July: Gone Fishing

Any time a staff member performs a great service, clients and staff are invited to write that person's name on a fish-shaped paper and put it in a fish bowl at the front desk.

The Plan

Create signage at the front desk explaining the contest and have fish decorations. Announce the winners at the staff meeting.

The Reward (all staff)

Bragging rights! Plus, a fishing trip getaway or a hotel stay is always a great getaway. This is where your staff can choose what works for their life style.

■ ■ ■

August: Polish Predictions

Give nail-polish purchasers a chance to win nail products and services by correctly guessing the number of polishes in a bowl.

The Plan

Instead of discarding last season's half-full bottles of nail polish, you fill a huge glass bowl with them. Post a big sign at the front desk explaining the promotion. For every purchase of one polish at the regular price, clients are asked to guess the number of polishes in the bowl. Whoever guesses correctly wins a free manicure and pedicure.

The Reward (all staff)

Each guest is worth 1 point. When a staff member earns 10 points, he or she is invited to go to lunch with (and on) the boss! Never underestimate the simple act of spending one-on-one time with your team.

■ ■ ■

September: Back to School

As kids go back to school, encourage clients to take advantage of increased free time by pampering themselves with additional salon and spa services.

The Plan

When a client adds on additional services to his or her preexisting appointment, he or she will receive 10 percent off of that day's services.

The Reward (all staff)

Each additional service is worth 1 point. Each staff member needs to get at least 10 guests per week to add services. Not only will this earn additional monies in service sales, but for every 10 points, the staff member would earn a complimentary service for himself or herself. Just because staff members work there does not mean they will make time to get services there. Too many times, we find people in the industry forget how it is to be a client. By having your staff get services, you may find it is a true win-win.

■ ■ ■

October: Giving

"Giving" is a gift-certificate program designed to encourage your clients to purchase gift certificates to help with the craziness of the holiday shopping time.

The Plan

Clients who purchase at least $50 in gift certificates will receive a complimentary gift. The gift could be 15 percent off retail products, 10 percent off a new service, or, if you need to get rid of old products on your shelves that just will not sell, wrap them up as gift sets and give them to your clients who purchase at least $50 in gift certificates. Once you have chosen what your gift is going to be, stick with it and talk it up! Encourage your clients to give gift certificates and give ideas of who might like to receive one (bosses, in-laws, babysitters, etc.).

The Reward (all staff)

Create an incentive for your team. The reward for hitting their retail goal could be more time off during the holiday season or getting an awesome gift. What does your team want? Ask!

■ ■ ■

November: In the Box

Offer a client referral program. The winning client with the most referrals wins a year's worth of fine services.

The Plan

Clients are given referral cards. When the referred client visits, he or she drops the referral card into the ballot box with the referring client's name on it. The more referrals, the more times the client's name goes into the ballot box, increasing the client's chances to win.

The Reward (all staff)

For every referral a staff member's client gives, the staff member receives 2 points. To receive a completion stamp, the staff member needs to have 60 points. If the staff member gets 5 referrals per week, this would bring in 20 new guests.

■ ■ ■

December: Wrapping the Year Up! (Christmas, Hanukkah, Kwanza)

Gift certificates, gift sets, and gifts of all kinds that can be used as "stocking stuffers" go well; this is also the season to empty the shelf of all the merchandise you have had on your shelves for too long. If you are going to have a sale, now is the time. You can gift-wrap the items at no extra charge if purchases are made before the client's appointment. What better way to have him or her wait on those December days? Specialty items for all should be stocked during this month and could include curling irons, brushes, and candles.

The Plan

The goal is to sell through all gift sets and/or a predetermined dollar amount of gift certificates.

The Reward

Determine what the reward will be in November; make it as fun and exciting as you can. Give the team an opportunity to voice what they would like to receive as a reward. (Remember, you have the last say, and it must work for all parties. You are in business to make a profit.)

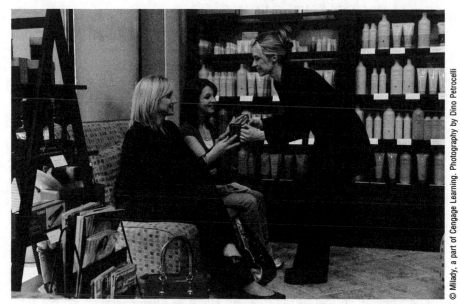

Most of the promotion of services and retail items is done on a personal basis in the salon and spa.

MARKETING RETAIL ITEMS

You have probably noticed that most of the promotion of services and retail items is done on a personal basis in the salon and spa. Newspaper ads, while good, are no substitute for personal selling. The more personal an approach, such as cards through the mail and/or e-mail, a telephone call, or talking directly to a group, the better.

Specialty Items

The sale of clothing and/or jewelry should be done in a separate area. Hair spray that floats in the air can ruin good clothing in a matter of days. Also, fine jewelry should be placed where it can be watched at all times and the inventory count maintained (a few salons and spas do combine the areas, but most of the time, it does not meet with much success). You may find that in most cases, technicians are not interested in this type of thing and will not promote it well. One way to test this for your salon and spa is to consider having specialty items carried only under consignment.

■ IMPORTANT RULES

When merchandising in a salon and spa, keep the following in mind:

1. Know your customer.
2. Know what you are selling.
3. Know who is going to sell it.
4. Know how much it costs and what kind of profit you intend to make.

At the end of the year, be sure to evaluate what you have sold and profits made from such sales. Then plan another sales program and carry it through.

Chapter 9 Summary

- A salon and spa must launch and maintain an active program to get new customers in and retain them as customers.

- The three steps in merchandising are getting the customer into the salon and spa, giving customers what they want, and selling customers what they need.

- All purchasing of back-stock items and retail items should be done by one person. Choosing a retail line is a very important decision; a good distributor can help with promotions and education.

- To merchandise in a salon and spa, know your customers, know what you are retailing, know who will retail it, and know your costs and what kind of profit you will make.

Review Questions

1. What is the difference between gross sales and real profit?

2. How can a meeting or training seminar be used to help stylists increase their business?

3. How can "establishing a time line" during the consultation help a technician deliver great *service* and *satisfaction* to the client?

4. What can a technician say and do to ensure the return of a client who does not rebook at the end of an appointment?

5. List three things that you should consider when designing a promotion.

Use of Cosmetology Schools by Salons and Spas

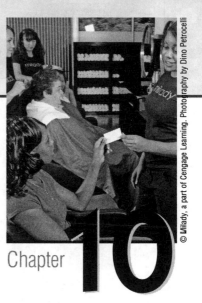

Chapter 10

Many salon and spa owners and managers, as well as technicians, overlook one of the most important factors in their careers: staying current with the times. Clients can and do change salons and spas and technicians. According to current statistics, the average client will stay with you three to five years. Clients leave for numerous reasons, but the greatest reason is indifference—meaning that you do not care enough to treat them differently. Year after year, it is the same redundant looks. Remember, it is like wearing your favorite shirt day after day—even though you feel great in it, you would eventually become bored with it. In the business of customer service, it is important to be aware of what causes your clients to change salons and spas and/or technicians. Since we are in the business of fashion, your clients are looking to your professional guidance to inspire the latest fashions versus getting the same look. If we are not aware of the current trends, how do we expect our clients to trust that our knowledge is valuable? One of the excuses voiced by most technicians is that some clients "cannot wear the new styles." Sometimes, this is true. For the most part, however, clients are looking for a hairstyle that is different, becoming, and up-to-date. Those in the salon and spa industry need to search out educational resources actively to keep with the changing times and trends.

To keep up to date, a technician must practice the new techniques of hairstyling and haircutting. Unfortunately, not all technicians have time during the course of a busy day to experiment with untried and unproven hairstyles. Good cosmetology schools, on the other hand, have the time to experiment with new styling techniques. Trained instructors stand ready to assist the willing technicians with styling

125

in the latest trends. These instructors make a business of creating hairstyles that keep up with the trends.

Several education classes are offered each year. Some states require continuing-education classes to keep your license—these may be referred to as **CEU credits**—while others do not. However, it is highly recommended that, regardless of state laws, you further your education. Licensed cosmetology schools do offer one advantage: a chance to practice and experiment under supervision on mannequins and human models. Besides hairstyling classes, cosmetology schools offer classes in advanced haircutting and coloring techniques, permanent waving, salon and spa management, and so much more.

CEU credit
Continuing-education classes to keep a professional license.

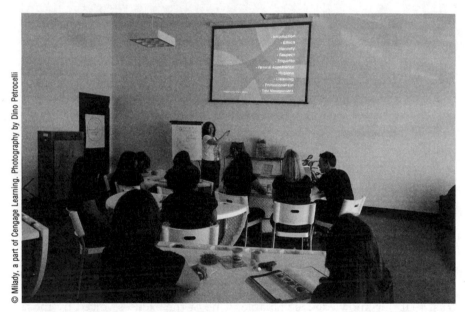

These instructors make a business of creating hairstyles that keep up with the trends.

SPECIALIZED STUDY

Specialized studies in the beauty industry are offered in most cosmetology schools. One of the most important factors to remember is that spas and salons dictate what the schools offer for classes. No different than the days of Vidal Sassoon, Where in 1963, Sassoon created short, geometric haircuts that consumers could blow dry and style out themselves at home. Consumers and salons and spas were demanding precision haircutting. As a result, Vidal Sassoon was a key force in commercializing precision haircutting in their schools, and other schools across the country soon followed the same direction. Salons and spas and schools need to be in partnership with one another to better serve the public. A school cannot offer courses in what a salon and spa needs if the school is unaware of what those needs are. It is important for both schools and salons and spas to have open communication, and to communicate with one another on a regular basis.

More recently, trends that have occurred are hair extensions, microdermabrasion, and lash extensions, to name a few. Many schools have classes in general that are in their curriculum, but they are not always offered. These schools also offer your basic foundation classes, such as color, cuts, and perms, not to mention products.

In the last decade, many schools have become product-driven. In these particular schools, the students are heavily trained on product knowledge. These include Redkin, Paul Mitchell, and Aveda schools, just to name a few. The benefit of these schools for the salon and spa is that your future employees should be well-versed in these product lines upon entering your business, enabling the salon and spa to cut the cost and time of training new employees. Remember that all schools offer product knowledge that is an asset to your business. Retail is a large profit center for the salon and spa and therefore should be considered when looking for potential employees.

One of the benefits of taking these specialized courses is that they offer additional sources of income for the salon and spa and set you apart from your competitors. If a salon and spa pays for special classes, the salon and spa can deduct it from its income tax as an expense. If the technician pays for special classes, he or she will get a tax break. Travel, hotel bills, food, and all expenses associated with the class are considered part of the class.

Salons and spas may use the schools for both employment and information. Who better knows the latest laws and requirements for salons and spas and students than the schools? Most schools are more than willing to share their knowledge of the industry with salon and spa owners and technicians.

■ EMPLOYMENT SERVICES

Each year, thousands of salons and spas across the country are looking for good, qualified technicians to fill vacancies created by technicians who have left the industry for various reasons. Some reasons include moving, family, opening their own salon and spa, or leaving the industry. Regardless of the reason, the important thing to remember is that this is your business, and you need to be proactive versus reactive. Your salon and spa must be ever alert for new talent to replace technicians who have left.

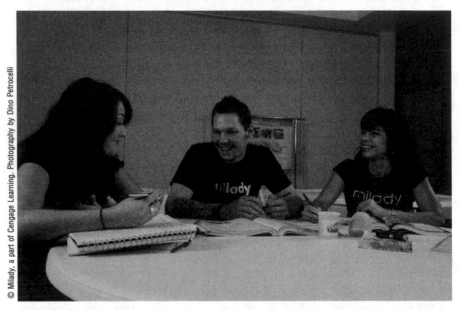

The easiest and most accessible place to look for new talent is your local cosmetology school.

Cosmetology schools furnish a service in this area. Each year, schools turn out technicians of every type to fit the needs of any salon and spa. When you need a new employee, first call the local cosmetology school and state your needs. Most schools are happy to assist in helping an employer obtain the right technician. One of the important factors is to establish a working relationship with the cosmetology schools. This can be easily done in numerous ways:

- Visiting the schools
- Teaching specialty classes at the school
- Participating in job fairs
- Offering tours of your salon and spa
- Leave service menus, brochures, and flyers at the school
- Offering discounts to teachers and students at your salon and spa

The bottom line is: Do not be the best-kept secret around; do your best to make those around you take notice.

Just like your salon and spa is trying to be noticed by the schools, the students are being noticed by their instructors. The cosmetology schools and instructors have daily contact with their students for several months. Who better knows about their personality, their customer relations, their cooperation, their attitude, their styling ability, their promptness, their willingness, and their telephone approach? Simply put, you are hiring a personality and training a skill, and a call to the cosmetology school will aid in making your selection.

■ INFORMATION CENTERS

At one time or another, technicians, salon and spa owners/managers have problems. They can be managerial or technical. In either case, a good school with a well-trained, up-to-date staff can help solve some of them or can provide information about where the answer may be found. Here are the most common reasons to use a school (you may also contact your State Board for this information):

- Employment services
- Continuing-education classes
- The current state licensing requirements
- **Reciprocity** (find out if there are other requirements for licensing)
- Sanitation and sterilization laws

Other information often obtainable from beauty schools includes:

- Product information (color, permanent waves, relaxers, retail products, etc.)
- Price schedules for an area
- Types of salons in the area
- Styling trends
- Corrective procedures
- Management procedures

reciprocity
Interaction between two parties for mutual advantage. For example, a hairstylist may be moving from one state to another and will require a new license. Some states will transfer those hours while others will require additional hours or testing out before being issued a license in that state.

The officer who usually handles this type of information is the school owner or director. If you need technical information, the instructors specializing in the various subjects will be most helpful.

Your ability to work with schools will depend upon the degree of mutual respect that has built up between salons and spas and schools in your community.

Chapter 10 Summary

- Keeping up to date and adapting modern trends by furthering your education will keep your clients from changing salons and stylists.

- Retail is a large profit center, and therefore should be considered when looking for potential employees.

- A good cosmetology school has a well-trained, up-to-date staff that can help your salon and spa with the hiring process.

- Use the schools for questions and challenges regarding employment services, licensing requirements, and product information.

Review Questions

1. If a technician is sure that a client would not be interested in changing his or her style to be more in line with current trends, why should he or she still conduct a thorough consultation?

2. How do salons and spas influence schools? How does a partnership between the two better serve the public?

3. What helpful information can a cosmetology instructor give an employer? Discuss at least five personality traits or habits that they may have observed.

4. What could you do as an employer to maintain a working relationship with the cosmetology schools in your area? Discuss in detail at least two ways that you could be involved with the school.

Labor-Related Laws

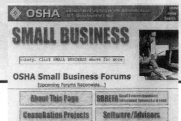

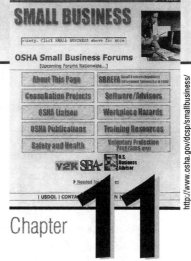

Chapter **11**

There are over 400 federal laws, thousands of state laws, and several thousand local regulations that pertain to employees' rights and hiring practices. The intention of this chapter is to provide an overview of these. As you embark on the adventure of becoming a business owner, you should always consult an attorney in employment law in your state or local community for laws governing your salon and spa's business. This chapter is not intended to be used as a law reference, but rather to provide a salon and spa owner with a core understanding of laws that are currently in place.

Lawsuits are prevalent in today's society. Lawsuits can be brought against any employer for any reason if the employee feels it is justified. Laws are formed in these ways. First, the local, state, or federal legislative structure, meeting in regular or special sessions, can pass a law that governs an industry or special segment of society. These laws may or may not be constitutional, but remain in force until challenged. The court system will rule on each law or section of the law as lawsuits surface. This has the effect of confirming the law or defining certain aspects of the law. Laws that have withstood the court action are stronger than those that have not.

The second way a law is formed is by **legal action** brought by one person against another or a corporation. This is a costly and time-consuming process. When a court renders a judgment, others can use this judgment as a form of legal leverage to settle disputes.

The third way a law is formed is by the vote of the people on an issue. Again, these laws are subject to legal review by the court system and may be found to be constitutional or unconstitutional. Each city and township has several "laws" passed by the voters that regulate everything from what is a public nuisance to the activities of business.

Lawsuit

A civil action brought before a court of law in which the plaintiff claims to have received damages from a defendant's actions and is now seeking a legal or equitable remedy.

For salon and spa owners, laws governing the practice of cosmetology and barbering are usually controlled by the state legislators, with specific items left to the State Board of Barbers and Cosmetologists to regulate actual practice or activities of the trade. These specific items are known as *rules and regulations*.

Labor laws do not generally speak to cosmetologists and barbers directly, but form guidelines for all businesses to follow. **Labor laws** for the most part came out of the 1960s, with actions targeted to stop segregation and discrimination. In short, these laws were to give all members of society an equal opportunity for employment regardless of race, color, or ethnic background. Later, the categories of gender and people with disabilities were added to the protected groups. Local communities often went a step further to introduce laws against discrimination because of sexual orientation, age, language, physical disabilities, mental disabilities, dress, height and weight, drug and alcohol usage, and so forth. All this effort was to govern the labor force and its practices.

Usually, businesses with fewer than five employees are exempt from **federal labor laws**. The federal government usually deals with laws that are meant to govern businesses with 15 to 25 employees or businesses that conduct business across state boundaries. State laws and local laws may govern businesses with as few as one or two employees. Some guidelines are given here with reference material and documents to follow. Remember to consult your labor lawyer to obtain specifics for your area.

■ GUIDELINES FOR OWNERS/MANAGERS

1. *Treat all employees equally.* All salon and spa documents can be given in a hard copy or electronically. You will find that an electronic copy cuts costs. Basic information needed spells out hours to be worked, vacation schedules, compensation for work, customer relations, dress/uniform policies, cleanup duties, days off, and so forth; these must be fair to all employees and consistent with the years of service to the salon and spa and related duties. Therefore, a policy document shows that all employees are treated the same regardless of age, sex, sexual orientation, marital status, religion, or nationality, and applies to all employees equally.

2. When marketing for a salon and spa position, be sure that *discriminatory statements are not used*. "Male only," "must be single female," and "must be under 25 years old" have been outlawed by laws and court rulings.

3. When interviewing, be careful not to ask questions or make statements that could be perceived as discrimination. Questions such as, "That is a fine cross you are wearing; do you go to a local church?" and "What does your husband do for a living?" do not relate to the job and are illegal to ask in a job interview. These forms of questioning may lead to a lawsuit.

4. You have a right to have the interviewee take a skill test for the position. However, make sure all applicants are scored on all items required for the job. A male technician must do a facial or manicure if you require all female technicians to do a facial and manicure.

5. The compensation (pay and benefits) for the employee must be the same at each level of employment. You may pay employees of 10 years with the business a greater amount than a new hire; however, all employees of the same level must be compensated at the same rate.

6. The compensation for all employees must be the same, and the benefit package must be the same. However, you may be able to offer different compensation packages if the true value of the compensation is the same.

Example:
$200 each month is awarded as "**flex dollars**." They can be used to purchase health insurance, dental insurance, babysitting services, and so forth. The primary requirement is that all employees get $200 in flex dollars, which they can spend as they see fit.

flex dollars
A term used to assign values to employees benefits.

7. All forms of advancement must be the same for all employees. If you offer advanced styling classes, they must be offered to all employees. If you send one stylist to a special training seminar, you must offer to send them all. You can send them at different times and to different places, but the opportunity must be made available to all and should cost the same amount.

8. Shoptalk is necessary and healthy to promote good working relationships among employees. However, if the conversation becomes offensive to one individual, it should stop.

9. Keep all employee records confidential and all employee applications and interview forms confidential. All such records and forms are usually required to be held for a period of time, and most can be electronically stored.

Regardless of how hard you try not to break any of the labor and employment laws, chances are you are breaking some or bending some without knowing it. Insurance can be purchased to cover the salon and spa owner and management personnel against judgments resulting from any legal suits brought by employees. Avoid at all cost any actions that could be viewed as *deliberately, intentionally, or willfully prejudicial* when dealing with one employee over another or one job candidate over another.

For an employee or a potential employee to receive damages from a salon and spa or management, several items must be proven. All states have different rules. Always consult a good labor attorney if a case is brought against you and your company.

■ INTERVIEW NO-NOS

The goal in a job interview is to build a friendly rapport with the candidate while abstracting important and valuable information. During the interview process, there are questions that may cross boundaries of what is legal to ask. To protect yourself and your business from any legal trouble and/or embarrassment, know which questions to avoid while still being able to get to the root of the questions.

The following two questions illustrate the difference between legal and illegal wording.

> "Do you plan to have children?" (This question is *illegal*.) Clearly, the concern here is that family obligations will get in the way of work hours. Instead of asking about or making assumptions about family situations, get to the root of the issue by asking directly about the candidate's availability.
>
> "Are you available to work evenings and weekends, on occasion? Can you travel for educational classes?" (This question is *legal*.) While some salons and spas are small operations and have fewer than five employees, they still might come under federal and state guidelines for employment practices. This is especially true if the salon and spa is a member of a large national or state chain. The rule here is "Better safe than sorry."

■ MAJOR LAWS AFFECTING THE COSMETOLOGY INDUSTRY

The laws stated here are the major federal laws that have a direct effect on businesses employing over 15 people or who do business across state borders. Copies can be found in local libraries, from the U.S. Government Printing Office, and on the Web. A review of them will give you some insight into labor law.

The Civil Rights Law of 1964

This law deals with discrimination based on race, sex, and religious beliefs. It later was expanded through the Occupational Qualification Act to include age, national origin, disabilities, and marital status. The wording that keeps surfacing throughout the legal literature is that employers must not discriminate when hiring and must make *reasonable accommodations* to support those who are employed. This can be as simple as allowing a person to be absent from work on certain religious holidays. It does not require that the employer pay the wages of a person who is absent unless holidays of other groups are paid. In that case, all employees must be treated equally.

The Pregnancy Discrimination Act of 1978

This provides leave time to *pregnant employees or their spouses*. It allows time for female employees to go to and from doctor's appointments, have various medical tests, and take time off for delivery and care of the newborn. The male employee is afforded the same benefit. The reasoning, besides equal treatment under the law, is that he may have to provide transportation, medical assistance, child care, meals, and so forth to his wife and children during this time. The employer does not have to provide financial assistance for time lost unless sick leave is requested during this period. The law does not state that the same job, in the same facility, with the same equipment, with the same compensation and scheduling, be provided when the employee returns.

Something to consider: Is it the employer's responsibility to provide time and a place to breast-feed a newborn or a place to house the infant during working hours? Normally the answer is no; however, if you allow one employee to do so, you must offer all employees the same right.

The Age Discrimination Act of 1978

The Age Discrimination Act of 1978 deals with hiring people over 40 years old. It is fairly straightforward in the beauty and barber trade. If all employees must cut a head of hair in 20 minutes as a requirement of employment, and it takes another employee longer, this may be a reason to eliminate a candidate for a position. The employer is put in a position of having to prove that an employee who is slow due to age is causing loss of income and would put the business in financial trouble. This is extremely difficult to prove because the new employee candidate has no track record for customer service in that salon and spa. When in doubt, do not violate the law.

The Immigration Reform and Control Act of 1986

This law prohibits the employment of illegal aliens, except under certain conditions. The main issue here is to make sure that the employer has a valid license in the state in which the establishment is located and has legal papers allowing any aliens to have employment within the United States. Should the government question the employment of an individual, the burden of proof falls upon the employer. Thus, copies of all papers for an individual are a must. A good rule of thumb is: When in doubt, check first with the Department of Labor within your state.

The Americans with Disabilities Act of 1990

The Americans with Disabilities Act of 1990 (ADA) and the Rehabilitation Act of 1994 have defined various illnesses or disabilities in a very broad format. While the federal laws deal with operations of 15 or more people, some state and local laws apply to all businesses regardless of the number of employees.

The current definition of disabilities includes—along with obvious disabilities (loss of limbs, sight, hearing, ability to walk, etc.)—obesity, suicidal tendencies, borderline personalities, post-traumatic stress syndrome, diabetes, allergies to tobacco and chemicals, HIV/AIDS, alcoholism, and drug addictions, all falling under the ADA.

The law requires employees to make *reasonable* accommodations to disabled applicants. This may include ramps for wheelchairs, removal of decorative barriers, purchase of furniture that helps the disabled, and special equipment such as telephones, lighting fixtures, toilet facilities, and so forth. However, a situation in which an employee has the ability to generate $40,000 in sales, but accommodating that employee would require remodeling that would cost $100,000 with no guarantee that he or she would stay with the company for a period of time, would probably be found to be excessive.

▪ WAGES AND HOURS

The Fair Labor Standards Act (FLSA) standardizes wages and overtime pay in most public and private employment. The act requires employers to pay employees the federal minimum wage and overtime pay of 1.5 times the regular rate of pay, unless employees are otherwise exempt.

EMPLOYMENT CONTRACTS

Employment contracts have been tested in state and local courts across the country. They require a prospective employee to sign a contract in which the applicant agrees to work for a company for a given amount of time for a given compensation equal to or significantly less than other employees. Usually, the decrease in compensation is for marketing, promotions, and education that the salon and spa is willing to provide the new employee. This is to give the business a chance to recoup the cost of hiring a new employee. These costs are usually the cost of marketing, guaranteed wage, training, uniforms, and so forth. In the contract, the new employee agrees not to work for another salon and spa within a certain number of miles or for a period of time after the employment has ended.

Contract dispute court cases have favored both the employer and the employee. In cases where the employer has received damages, it was normally for profits from a technician's service based on average income generated by the technician until the end of the contract. The salon and spa had to show actual costs incurred on behalf of the employee since the start of the contract and those activities related only to that employee.

> **Example:**
> The employee was paid to go to a training class to further her skills, but no one else was paid to attend a class that year.

If all technicians were paid to go to the education classes, this cost would not apply. To win this case, the employer's records must be specific to the contracted employee only. The employee, to win this case, must show that the contract kept the person from gaining employment in a reasonable fashion.

> **Example:**
> In a small town of four salons and spas, each of which is less than 2 miles apart, there is a restriction of a 7-mile radius for working in another salon and spa.

This would eliminate employment in that town for all employees who signed and agreed to the contract. The time limit placed on the

employment contract
A traditional written agreement that is signed and agreed to by employer and employee.

individual before employment in another salon and spa is acceptable is another area of concern. The employee may have agreed not to perform any salon and spa services for a certain period of time after this contract in any location except in the business with which the contract is in force. Usually, a judge will allow the person to work pending the trial on this contract, which may take several years to get into the courtroom. This virtually voids the contract except for the fact that the technician may have to pay for training and other compensation parts of the contract.

Note: The cost of litigation is extremely expensive. The attorneys usually wish to be paid on an "as-we-go" basis. So, you could spend several thousands of dollars in attorney fees, filing fees, recording fees, court fees, and so forth, and never get any return on your lawsuit. This is true for both the employee and the employer. The time required for these suits to come to trial is also very long. During this time, the technician may have left town, may have gotten married, or may be no longer working, or may be employed in another occupation, all of which will affect the outcome of the trial.

Chapter 11 Summary

- Employer's can be sued for anything at any time provided the employee feels that some damage has been caused to him or her emotionally, financially, professionally, or physically.

- An increasing number of communities are adopting laws protecting employees from unfair business practices. Most of these have been based on federal laws, but normally relate to businesses with 1 to 25 employees.

- While interviewing and conducting business, be sure that the business does not have employees, managers, or owners using practices that could be construed as deliberately, intentionally, or willfully prejudicial.

- The Americans with Disabilities Act of 1990 and the Rehabilitation Act of 1994 now form the basis for most labor disputes with regard to employment practices. Before you act, read these laws carefully, especially with regard to the definition of who is considered disabled.

- *Reasonable accommodation* must be followed in making a salon and spa accessible to all employees. The salon and spa should not be held responsible for such accommodations to the extent of extreme financial stress.

- Contracts for employment are used in many areas of employment; those that have been tested have resulted in mixed reviews. All contracts should be reviewed by your lawyer, as they will be the ones to represent you and your business if a lawsuit is filed.

Review Questions

1. What must you remember if you require a skill test as part of the interview process?

2. List two reasons why the Pregnancy Discrimination Act of 1978 provides leave time not only for female employees but for male employees also.

3. How would you describe a *reasonable* accommodation to a disability applicant as opposed to an *excessive* accommodation?

4. What does the Fair Labor Standards Act require of employers?

5. What are the strengths and weaknesses of using employment contracts in salons? List at least one of each.

Salon and Spa Personnel

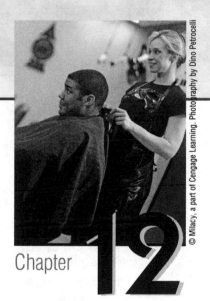

Chapter **12**

After you have selected your salon and spa type, named it, secured the **lease agreement**, hooked up to public utilities, chosen the décor, equipment, and supplies, and selected and/ or created all your **policies and procedures**, your next thought should be selecting and securing the right staff.

Almost everything in your salon and spa business depends upon the competency of your employees; therefore, the people you hire and the way in which you train them are critical to your success. The idea is to find employees who are going to earn their wages, not just collect them.

Hiring individuals with good personalities and good work ethics truly can increase your sales. **Customers** feel more comfortable, secure, and happy when someone who is friendly and capable is aiding them. The **employee** becomes even more important if you add retail merchandise to your salon and spa.

FINDING GOOD EMPLOYEES

You may already know one or more technicians with whom you wish to build your business. However, most salons and spas must at some point run an ad in the local newspaper, advertise on the Internet, or visit cosmetology schools for securing additional staff to service a growing clientele. Here are a few suggestions for doing just that.

Advertise in a Newspaper

One of the most common ways to find technicians is to place a newspaper advertisement. However, in order to attract the type of people you want to hire, you will want to stipulate your high standards in

lease agreement
A contract by which the landlord (or lessor) gives the tenant (or lessee) the use and possession of lands, buildings, property, and so forth, for a specified time and in return for fixed payments.

policies and procedures
A set of documents that describe the business's policies for operation and the procedures designed to fulfill the policies

customers
Also known as a *client, guest, or purchaser*; a current or potential buyer or user of the products and services provided by the business.

141

employee
A person who is hired to provide services to a company on a regular basis in exchange for compensation and who does not provide these services as part of an independent business.

résumé
A marketing tool used by individuals to secure a new job; contains a summary of relevant job experience and education.

Internet ad
Online marketing, a form of promotion that uses the World Wide Web for the express purpose of delivering marketing messages to attract customers.

search engines
Web sites that search for information on the World Wide Web. The searches are presented in a list form and the results are often called "hits."

the ad. Mention that you are seeking an inside sales person with flexible hours in a pleasant, business atmosphere.

Place the ad in the "Help Wanted, Professional" section. If the first word is either a headline or capitalized—for example, "Hair Stylist"—your ad has a better chance of being read by prospective staff. Obviously, the larger and more elaborate your ad, the more response you can expect. Be sure, however, that your ad matches the possibilities available in your salon. Placing the name of the salon and spa in the ad will give recognition to your salon and spa. Remember always to include your contact information, whether it is an e-mail address or a fax or phone number. This will enable prospective technicians/employees to send a **résumé** or fill out an application prior to an interview so that you may screen them. This will ultimately save you valuable time in the selection process.

Advertise on the Web

In today's world, most potential employees are surfing the Web. One of the easiest and most productive ways to find technicians is to place an **Internet ad**. This will give you a larger pool of potential candidates. This can be accomplished through **search engines** and industry-related sites. For example, you may want to place an ad through craigslist.com or salonemployment.com.

Using search engines to place "sponsored ads" means that when people search one of your keywords, your ad will appear next to the search results. Potential employees simply click your ad to learn more about your available openings. You are advertising to an audience that is already interested.

You will want to include the same type of information in your Internet ad that you would in your newspaper ad; however, you may take the opportunity to be more detailed in your job description (you will not be charged per letter as in the newspaper). Also, be aware that some Internet ads must be refreshed frequently in order to keep the ad current.

Visit a Cosmetology School

Most schools are more than happy to assist in helping an employer obtain the right technician. Schools turn out students of every type to fit the needs of any salon and spa. You will never have a better opportunity to be in front of a more captive audience than you will by visiting your local schools. One of the most important factors is to establish a working relationship with the cosmetology schools. It is not enough just to ask the school to send a potential employee to you; you must be proactive by contacting them. For more detailed information on using cosmetology schools, refer to Chapter 10.

Note: Employees have been known to quit without warning, so when you come across someone you like and he or she expresses an interest in working for you, take his or her name and number and begin a file. Then, it will be easier to find the right person without going to the trouble of advertising for a new technician when you need one.

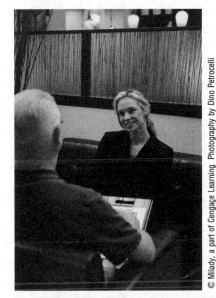

Allow potential employees to do some of the talking.

THE INTERVIEW

You want staff who are enthusiastic about clients and who understand that they are in the service industry. Their job will be about *serving* the client. In other words, it is not about them; it is about the clients they serve. You want staff who can work constructively with their fellow technicians. Make sure you go over your requirements and expectations; they must be perfectly clear from the beginning. A lack of communication is the most common source of problems in an employee–employer relationship. Prepare a written job description and emphasize selling retail items, as well as add-on services, as a primary responsibility. Allow potential employees to do some of the talking, because this is one of the best ways for you to get a feel for their personality and ideas.

For an example of an application form, see Chapter 13. Without an application form, the interview will wander around in circles, and questions that should be answered will be left unasked. During the interview, use the evaluation sheet to record additional information on the applicant's appearance and personality. For a sample of the evaluation sheet, see Chapter 13.

Using both of these sheets will help you to avoid the unwise hiring of undesirable personnel. It can cost the average salon and spa thousands of dollars in marketing, **sales promotion**, loss of clientele, and **additional salaries** before a new technician can make a profit for a salon and spa. Choose your salon and spa personnel wisely.

The information on the application form will help you pinpoint specific areas that you need to explore more fully during the interview. The questions you ask and how you ask them will help you elicit not just responses but attitudes. Be friendly. Avoid strong reactions to anything the applicant says. Above all, remember that the interview is a time for you to listen. One very sure sign of a potentially troublesome employee is the tendency to shift blame from the self to others. Of course, other people do create problems, but a resourceful, positive person assumes some responsibility for his or her own actions and always assumes that there is something he or she can do to improve the situation—without being destructive or hostile. "Bad-mouthing" the former employer or co-workers is a sign of a negative personality.

Here are some open-ended questions that will help you get a look at your prospective employee's attitudes and beliefs.

1. What do you like the best about working in a salon and spa?
2. Describe the best workday you ever had in a salon and spa.
3. What made that day such a good one?
4. Describe the ideal day of work in a salon and spa.
5. What do you find most challenging about being a technician?
6. What is the most difficult situation you ever had with a client?
7. How did you react?
8. How can such situations be avoided?
9. What makes a good co-worker?
10. What makes a bad co-worker?
11. What would you do if you were working next to a technician who had graduated with you from the same cosmetology school and now earns twice what you did?
12. What are your responsibilities to the salon and spa?
13. What are the salon and spa's responsibilities toward you?
14. What are your responsibilities toward your co-workers?

sales promotion
Activities, materials, and techniques used to support the marketing/sales efforts of the business.

additional salary
All income given over and above regular salary.

15. What are your co-workers' responsibilities toward you?
16. What are your responsibilities toward the clients?
17. What are the client's responsibilities toward you?
18. How does one solve problems with another person, boss, co-worker, or client?

◼ SETTING UP A PAY SCHEDULE

One of the most essential components of your job as a business owner is to figure out how much each of your staff members *should be* and *can be* paid. The amount you pay your technicians and **administrative staff—** management, front desk associates, and **assistants**—can make or break your salon and spa.

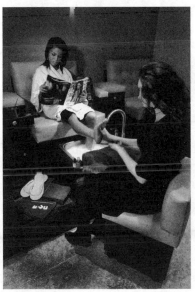

Typically, there are three ways to pay technicians.

How to Pay Your Technicians

Typically, there are three ways to pay technicians:

1. **Commission**
2. **Hourly/Salary**
3. **Booth rental**

administrative staff
Persons employed by the business owner who are hired to conduct daily business operations, such as a manager or front desk associate.

assistant
Within the beauty industry, a person who aids and supports beauty technicians; a technician in training.

commission
Revenue derived from services provided; paid to the technician performing those services.

hourly/salary
A compensation arrangement in which, in addition to an hourly wage, a periodic payment is given to the cosmetologist as income.

booth rental
System in which a renter leases space, or a "booth," within a salon and spa. The renter then uses the space to operate his or her own business for personal financial benefit, rather than for the success of the overall salon and spa.

Commission

Commissioned technicians are generally employees of the salon and spa. The technicians make a percentage of the money they make for services and products sold. The money they bring in, or do not bring in, directly affects your business. Since they are your employees, and they are not just renting from you, you have more of a say in how they conduct their affairs. You are responsible for the ins and outs of the day-to-day business—everything from scheduling to payroll to pricing, and so forth. Commission rates vary from one salon and spa to the next, but the average ranges are 42 percent to 50 percent. Any commission over 50 percent will no longer be bringing in a profit for your business. Commission on retail can also be paid, which generally runs between 5 percent and 15 percent. The technicians are paid entirely on the sales they bring to the business, allowing them to have greater control over their personal income.

Example:
A technician grosses $650 in a given period, with a rate of 40 percent.
$650 at 40% = $260
The technician receives a check for $260, less taxes.
In some cases, supplies are purchased by the technician, and a percentage is figured as a standard rate.

Example:
A technician sells two $45 hair colors and has general services of $82 in a given day. The cost of one tube of color to the technician is $5. The day's salary is figured as follows:

Hair color is $45 × 2 = $90, less cost ($5 × 2 = $10) =	$80
General services =	82
Total =	$162
Standard 50% =	81
Total day's pay =	$81

sliding percentage
Increasing or decreasing of a percentage of pay in accordance with a standard or a set of conditions normally designed to encourage staff productivity.

Another way of figuring wages is on a **sliding percentage**. Basically, this means that after reaching a certain gross sales figure, the percentage increases for the next block of sales. Usually, in the salon and spa industry, sales blocks are in increments of $100. A technician could typically make 40 percent on the first $100, 45 percent for the next $100, 50 percent for the next $100, and so forth, up to about 60 percent.

Example:
A technician brings in $850 during a pay period, and your salon and spa pays on a sliding percentage—40percent for the first

$300, 5 percent more for each $100 after that. The technician's wages would be:

$120 for the first $300
$45 for the next $100 (to $400)
$50 for the next $100 (to $500)
$55 for the next $100 (to $600)
<u>$150</u> for the rest ($250, the difference between $600 and $850)
$420 total wages

Hourly/Salary

As a salon and spa owner you may decide to pay your technicians an hourly or salary method. Many times a seasoned technicians feel there earnings are capped out because they are at the highest commission tier. In an hourly/salary based salon and spa you can still reward these people. Hourly/salary will allow you the freedom to reward the most deserving employees. Determining how to reward your employees can be based on a range of characteristics, from their skills in serving customers to their ability to work with other spa employees in a team environment. Keeping in mind that, that it is about rewarding and not punishing—singling out good behavior, not bad behavior. One way in which you can reward your employees in through profit-sharing.

Employee Benefits

Profit-Sharing

This plan is arranged so that all technicians, regardless of the time they have worked, receive the same percentage on their gross salary. After a given figure is reached, a certain amount of the profit is turned over to the employees in a **profit-sharing** program. The percentage of excess profit received is determined by an operator's gross total during the period.

profit-sharing
Various incentive plans that provide direct or indirect payments to employees that depend on the company's profitability, in addition to employees' regular salaries and bonuses.

Example:
A salon and spa sets a weekly gross of $1,000 before it starts profit-sharing. The profit-sharing is at the rate of 10 percent, paid on the gross of each technician. Technician A earns $600; Technician B earns $400; Technician C earns $200.

$1,200 less $1,000 leaves $200 on which the shop will pay in a profit-sharing program; 10 percent of $200 will be $20.

The profit may be split according to the gross of each technician.

Technician A—gross $600—6/12 of gross sales or 1/2
Technician B—gross $400—4/12 of gross sales or 1/3
Technician C—gross $200—2/12 of gross sales or 1/6

Profit sharing:

Technician A—1/2 times $20.00 = $10.00
Technician B—1/3 times $20.00 = $6.67
Technician C—1/6 times $20.00 = $3.33

These sums would then be added to the technicians' paychecks as an added income for working hard. One thing this system has built into it is a "help your neighbor" arrangement, since what your neighbor makes for the salon and spa may well increase your wages.

The profit-sharing plan described above in no way relates to the *pension-type profit-sharing plan* designed to produce retirement income. With this plan, payment is not paid to the employee, but to a fund that is reinvested to produce income.

This money, which is owned by the participant, is put aside without being taxed as income. Furthermore, earnings from this fund are not subject to income tax.

The monies involved are usually paid out when the employee leaves, dies, or retires. Payout arrangements vary according to how the plan is written. **Retirement plans** of any sort are of particular interest to those technicians who have a long-term perspective and want stability in their lives—very valuable employees. Vesting periods (the time it takes for an employee to earn 100 percent of the employer's contributions to the plan) encourage people to stay until fully vested, at least. However, such plans vary in complexity and appropriateness to your business, and funds can be invested with varying degrees of risk. Consult with a retirement-plan expert, and be sure that such a plan appeals to young employees.

Booth Rental

When you own a booth-rental salon and spa, you are the landlord, not the business owner. Each technician pays a rental fee for his or her station/room at an agreed-upon rate. This rate may be paid out on a daily, weekly, or monthly basis. Technicians are responsible for the day-to-day running of their own booths; they make their own appointments and set their own hours. The technicians are their own business owners. The **landlord** does not control pricing, quality, hours worked, or **customer service**. Booth-renters are responsible for doing their own taxes.

retirement plan
A special savings account, such as a 401(k) or Roth IRA, where an employee either defers part of his or her current income into a tax shelter, where it will grow tax-free until the employee withdraws it, or makes contributions into the account from after-tax income, where any gains on the principal are tax-free.

landlord
The owner of lands, buildings, property, and so forth that are rented or leased to an individual or business, called the *tenant.*

customer service
A series of activities created to improve the level of customer satisfaction. "Exceed customer expectation."

Example:

Mr. Jones owns a salon and spa. One of the stylists rents a booth for $200 a week. The stylist makes $400 in gross sales. Mr. Jones receives $200 in the form of **rent**, and the stylist receives $200 as a gross profit. Note that no taxes of any kind are deducted. Thus, the burden of taxes and bookkeeping now fall on the stylist.

A salon and spa owner who enters into a booth-rental agreement is truly a landlord in every sense of the word; however, he or she runs a substantial risk. While free of the need to keep records for the renters, to purchase supplies, and to supervise operations, the opportunity for gain is substantially reduced. Lacking the direction provided by a single owner/manager, the salon and spa's clientele may grow haphazardly. Lacking an identity, the salon and spa will have difficulty attracting a particular type of client.

Furthermore, state or federal taxing authorities may decide that the business is not truly a **rental agreement** if the owner exercises too much control over his or her renters—effectively treating them as employees—in which case the owner becomes liable for back taxes and penalties. These can be ruinously high. Abuse of the subcontractor relationship (which is how the government views booth rental) has led to intense scrutiny of any such operation. Because the laws governing this are a patchwork of requirements, some of them painfully vague, the person entering into a booth rental agreement is running a very real risk. And, as many a businessperson has found out, the **IRS** has authority far beyond that of many government agencies, and decisions can seem arbitrary.

Note: It is possible to mix any combination of the earnings to get the form of salary structure you wish.

Example:

- **Salary + Commission**
- **Hourly + Bonuses**

WHEN SHOULD A TECHNICIAN TAKE A VACATION?

This is an age-old problem. For a new salon and spa, it is impossible to know for sure. As years progress, a client traffic pattern starts to form. Salons and spas in one area may have a large number of customers in the

rent
An agreed-upon payment made periodically by a tenant to a landlord for the use of space, a building, a business, an office, and/or other property.

rental agreement
A contractual arrangement between two parties where the landlord agrees to rent to the tenant for an agreed amount of time.

IRS
The Internal Revenue Service.

Salary + Commission
A compensation arrangement in which, in addition to salary, a percentage of the money made from the provision of services is given back to the cosmetologist as income.

Hourly + Bonuses
A compensation arrangement in which, in addition to an hourly wage, a percentage of the money made from the provision of services is given back to the cosmetologist as income when certain predetermined goals are obtained.

summer; others may be busiest in the winter (especially if it is a winter resort). In some areas, farming and harvesting schedules may have a definite effect on traffic flow. Whatever your traffic patterns are, you will want to plan vacations around them and have technicians available when you need them. Making sure to schedule your vacations during your off season.

Exceptions must be made; too many, however, will destroy your entire work schedule. Here is a typical business pattern for a salon and spa located in a medium-sized college town near a tourist area. The pattern reflects weekly and monthly volume in graph form, which gives information at a glance.

Note that business volume is concentrated in the months of June, July, and August. This is due to tourist influence in the area.

The drop in October is due to clients paying bills for their children's back-to-school supplies, clothes, shoes, and so forth. In other words, they are short on cash. Starting December 1, note the increase in business due to the Christmas holidays. This lasts through January and then drops until Easter (early April). May and September are reasonably good months due to activities at the university.

With this type of business pattern, technicians in this salon and spa should be made to schedule their vacations during October, early November, February, March, and early April. Each salon and spa is different, as is each community. To be able to chart this business pattern, you must keep records over several years.

If you program all your vacations in a row, with each technician taking a week or two at a time, it is possible to hire a new technician for this block of time. This newcomer, after working a vacation block, can sometimes build enough business to warrant full-time employment. This is a very effective way to bring in new talent without upsetting the rest of the technicians in the salon and spa.

Note: When allowing time off for vacations, a good rule of thumb is to have one technician off at a time. What you want to avoid is not having enough technicians to service your clients.

SETTING UP A DUTY LIST

Cleaning duties can be a touchy subject, so be sure to specify your expectations in the very beginning. Do not wait until after you have hired the person to explain that some cleaning duties are required. It is possible the person would not have been as interested in the job if he or she had known this and, if that is the case, concealing the fact will not make him or her any more receptive to it.

To keep a salon and spa running smoothly, you must set up a duty list, which assigns certain cleaning duties to each employee. The result

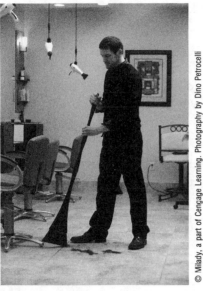

One of the most essential components is to figure out how much each of your staff members should and can be paid.

of such a list will be a clean, orderly, and attractive salon and spa. Employees should always clean equipment thoroughly after each use. The cleaning may sound simple, but you must emphasize that it needs to be done carefully and properly. Explain why it is necessary and what the possible consequences are if it is done improperly. Let your employees know that you expect them to keep their areas clean and well-organized; the front desk, for example, should be kept as tidy as possible since this usually is the first impression clients get when they enter the salon and spa. If it is messy or dirty, the client automatically will jump to the conclusion that the rest of the salon and spa is the same way.

Example:

A technician fails to clean her station and do her assigned duties. The cleaning person is then forced to spend an hour doing these duties (it takes her longer because she is unaware of where things go). The time that the cleaning person spends should, therefore, be paid for by the technician who made the mess. Her check would then read, "Gross salary—Taxes, etc.—Cleaning expense."

Here are some typical cleaning assignments given to technicians in smaller salon and spa having no full-time cleaning person:

1. Technicians will wash and dry their own styling chairs and styling stations each day.

2. Technicians will refill supplies kept in their stations/rooms at the end of each working day.

3. Technicians will clean all combs and brushes they use each day, unless otherwise directed.

4. Clean combs and brushes should be placed at the station at the end of each day (regardless of who does it).

5. Technicians should empty their own wastebaskets and wash them at the end of each day.

6. Technicians will replace any supplies or equipment taken from the supply room as soon as a service is completed.

7. Technicians will be assigned certain duties each day in some area of the salon and spa. These areas should be cleaned up and kept in an orderly fashion.

   Your duty is to _____.

8. Technicians will do their part to keep a designated area in the supply room neat.

   Your duty is to keep _____ clean and orderly.

■ SETTING UP A DRESS CODE AND GROOMING POLICY

Every salon and spa does need a dress code and grooming policy in writing to avoid any confusion of your expectations. The dress code for your salon and spa is up to the owner. If you are trying to portray an image of individuality in your salon and spa, your employees should do the same. You may want to set certain guidelines, like black pants and pastel shirts, just to keep the general image the same; however, you may find it is not necessary. Clothing can be fun, but should never be risqué. Also, keep in mind that it should be loose and comfortable enough to allow ease of movement. Below are examples of policies that may support you in making the decisions for your own business.

The hair of a technician should reflect the best workmanship of the salon and spa. All technicians should have their hair done at the salon and spa, not at a competitor's. The technicians should make arrangements to have their hair done before their first customer arrives, never while working on a client.

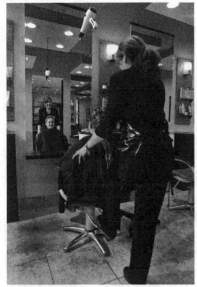

© Milady, a part of Cengage Learning. Photography by Dino Petrocelli

The dress code for your salon and spa is up to the owner.

Hair coloring should be encouraged, and the cost of such treatments should be paid to the salon and spa. If the salon and spa is selling wigs and hair goods, the technician should be encouraged to wear them at work. These should be sold to technicians at cost or slightly below to give added incentive for their purchase.

Makeup should be worn by all female employees. Remember that you are in the beauty industry, not working at the beach. There is such a thing as natural beauty, but in the retail industry, "You can't sell it if you don't wear it."

Today, tattoos and piercings have become popular. As the owner, you may want to include a policy on whether visible piercing and tattoos are appropriate or need to be covered up.

Daily bathing is necessary in our industry. A quick shower before coming to work, with some deodorant, works wonders. Daily teeth-brushing is also required. A male technician should shave each day. If a beard is worn, it should be trimmed daily and kept neat. Shoes should be clean and neat. At no time should a technician be allowed to work with dirty shoes or no shoes at all.

What does it look like, sound like, and feel like to your clients? Keep in mind: You are in the service business. Their view of you and your business matter.

▪ SEEING THROUGH YOUR CLIENTS' EYES

If you do not know what your clients are thinking, you need to find out. The best way to find out is to listen to what your clients are already telling you.

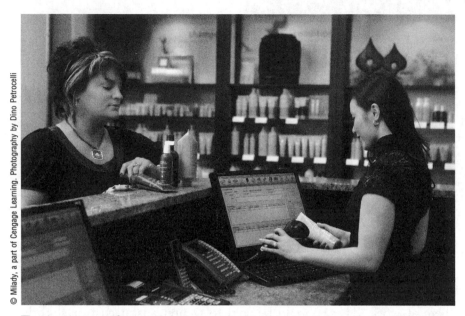

The best way to find out what your client is thinking is to try to see through her eyes and to listen to what she's telling you about her needs and wants as a client.

This can be done through a letter and questionnaire and gives the salon and spa a constant check on "how we are doing." The letter is general and asks the client for frank answers. This survey can be given to the client after the service, to be filled out immediately, or taken home with a stamped, self-addressed envelope. Surveys are also available through e-mail, which eliminates the cost of postage. The questionnaire does not require the client's signature.

Note: Take this opportunity to offer the client a reward for providing this information. The reward could come as a free travel-sized product or a 10 percent discount on a service.

After the questionnaire has been received by the owner/manager, he or she will then take all positive comments and share them with the entire staff. Any negative information received should be discussed in private with the employees involved. These are noted in the employee's personnel file.

Sample Letter and Questionnaire

We are in the business of making you feel good about your experience with us. Making sure you are satisfied and pleased is most important to us. Please help us provide you with the finest quality of service available by answering the questions below.

Place this in the drop box located at the front desk when you leave, or ask for a stamped, self-addressed envelope and mail it back at your convenience. We appreciate your response.

Did you find our service to be friendly, professional, and courteous when you called on the phone?	Yes	No
Were your questions regarding our services answered?	Yes	No
Was it easy to schedule your appointment?	Yes	No

Comments: _____
_____

Service:

Was the salon staff friendly and helpful?	Yes	No
Was your appointment taken on time?	Yes	No
Were you informed on how to continue your maintenance program on hair, skin, and nails at home?	Yes	No

Facilities:

How would you rate our salon and spa on:

Cleanliness?	Excellent	Good	Fair	Poor
Comfort?	Excellent	Good	Fair	Poor
Lighting?	Excellent	Good	Fair	Poor
Products?	Excellent	Good	Fair	Poor
Music?	Excellent	Good	Fair	Poor
Clothes/towel/robes, etc.?	Excellent	Good	Fair	Poor

Comments: _____
_____

Reasons for selecting our salon and spa:

Friend/Associate	Yellow pages	Newspaper
Magazine	Mailing	Gift certificate
Radio	Television	Noticed while driving by
Other		

| **Would you recommend the salon and spa to others?** | | Yes | | No |

Comments: _____

_____

| What is your overall impression of our salon and spa? | Excellent | Good | Fair | Poor |

How often do you visit the salon and spa?

Contact information:

It is our goal here at XYZ Salon and Spa to make sure your visit was most successful. Are there any other comments or suggestions you have? We would like to know.

Comments: _____

_____

Thank you for your time. Your comments make a difference.

Chapter 12 Summary

- In order to attract well-qualified people, you must have a well-run salon.

- Most salons and spas will at some time have to advertise in the newspaper, on the Internet, or with schools, and will have to interview prospective candidates.

- Above all, remember that the interview is a time for you to listen.

- There are three primary ways to compensate technicians: commission, hourly/salary, and booth rental.

- Vacation schedules, a duty list, and dress code and grooming policies should be clearly stated.

Review Questions

1. What are some of the differences between looking for new employees in the newspaper and looking for new employees on the Web? List at least three things that you want to consider before choosing the best way for you to advertise for salon and spa staff.

2. Why is it extremely costly to lose a technician? Discuss at least three ways in which it costs the salon and spa owner money to replace an employee.

3. Why might a technician be interested in working in a commission salon and spa instead of a salon and spa that pays an hourly wage?

4. How does a salon and spa duty list help to keep a salon and spa clean and appealing to clients? What can you do to keep technicians motivated to clean?

5. A list of recommendations for dress code and grooming are listed in the text. List the three that you believe are the most important and why you think they are so valuable.

Salon and Spa Forms and Items for Record-Keeping

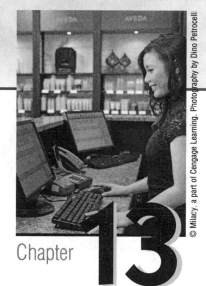

Chapter **13**

The forms you use in your salon and spa will determine whether you have on hand the information you need to run your business properly. Examples are provided in this book. Salon and spa education companies and trade magazines also sell forms kits and forms you will find useful in operating your business from day to day.

All computer-generated forms should be backed up in addition to keeping a hard copy on hand in case of computer failure or human failure from **accidental deletion**. Keep blank forms in a file marked "originals" so you can **photocopy** them should the need arise.

This is a starting point to develop your salon and spa's management information systems. As you see a need for additional information, you may wish to customize these forms to serve your particular salon and spa. Your **accountant/bookkeeper** will also have similar forms and related information available. A good accountant/bookkeeper can save the salon and spa time, effort, energy, and money because of his or her knowledge of the tax structure and tax requirements. With that in mind, to be in business and stay in business this information also needs to be easily accessible to you and you should be very familiar with it.

Regardless of how these forms are generated or become part of your computer system. In addition, you may want to have a hard copy (paper copy) available for a quick review. All reports are part of the daily operation of a business and should be updated on a daily basis.

Throughout this chapter are descriptions and examples of the types of forms you will need to conduct your daily operations.

accidental deletion
The unintended removal of client information, files, or documents.

photocopy
A photographic reproduction of any written, printed, or graphic material.

accountant
A practitioner of accountancy, who is licensed to practice the measurement, disclosure, or provision of assurance about financial statistics and information.

bookkeeper
A person who records the financial transactions of a person or business, including sales, purchases, income, and payments.

▪ EMPLOYEE APPLICATION FORMS

Your salon and spa should have some of these on hand. These forms can be stored in the desk file of the front desk associate and/or in the office. They need to be easily accessible. If your salon and spa has a Web site, the employee application form may also appear online. Prospective employees can fill out the application to be used by the salon and spa at a later date.

▪ EVALUATION AND INTERVIEW FORMS

These, like the application forms, need to be easily accessible, should be ordered in quantities of 100 or printed off your computer when your supply is down to 10, and should be upgraded as new ones are needed.

▪ APPOINTMENT BOOK

This is the most important record in your salon and spa. Be sure that this book is large enough to handle all technicians in your salon and spa. It should be bound with a cover, as it will be filed away as a permanent record of the salon and spa's activities.

Computerized appointment books should be backed up at the end of each day for income tax purposes. The information on all appointments for the next day should be printed out at the close of business the night before and backed up regularly in the event of a disaster such

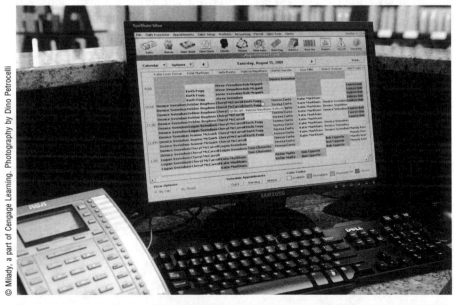

© Milady, a part of Cengage Learning. Photography by Dino Petrocelli

Appointment books can be either computerized or a physical, bound book.

EMPLOYEE APPLICATION FORM

Employee Application

Applicants are considered for all positions, and employees are treated during employment without regard to race, color, religion, sex, age, marital or veteran status, medical condition, or handicap.

Personal Information:

Name: _____ Name you would like to be called: _____

Current Address: _____
                    Street   City   State   Zip

Previous Address: _____
                    Street   City   State   Zip

Home Phone: _____ Cell: _____

Why do you feel you would be an asset to the XYZ Salon & Spa?
_____

Have you ever worked for a salon and spa before? _____ If yes, list locations, date, length of employment. _____
_____

If no, list your last two jobs with dates of employment:
_____
_____

Have you had advanced experience or training? _____
_____

If yes, please describe: _____

Where did you attend school?
_____

Have you held leadership positions in clubs organizations, civic groups, etc? If yes, briefly describe:
_____

What is your goal in life? _____

What are some of the things you would like to achieve during the next year?
_____

Why weren't you able to achieve this goal before?
_____

If you were to qualify for this opportunity, would any of the items below be a challenge? If so, why?
_____

A. Hours are from 8 a.m. to 8 p.m. _____
B. Working weekends _____
C. No personal telephone calls _____
D. No absenteeism _____
E. No tardiness _____
F. Training classes other than working hours _____

Are you looking for a career or a job? _____

Thank you for submitting an application. Please attach résumé if available.

EVALUATION SHEET
(for potential employees)

Name _____

Check the items in each category that seem most appropriate to the interview.

APPEARANCE
_____ well-groomed
_____ appropriate
_____ slovenly
_____ poor

COMMENTS _____

FACIAL EXPRESSION
_____ radiant
_____ thoughtful
_____ sullen
_____ happy
_____ solemn
_____ smiling

COMMENTS _____

HANDS AND FACE
_____ healthy appearance
_____ well cared for
_____ heavy makeup
_____ dirty

COMMENTS _____

APPROACH
_____ poised
_____ forward
_____ awkward
_____ timid

COMMENTS _____

ATTITUDE
_____ cooperative
_____ enthusiastic
_____ indifferent
_____ attentive
_____ arbitrary

COMMENTS _____

VOLUME OF VOICE
_____ too loud
_____ easily audible
_____ pleasant
_____ too low
_____ shrill

COMMENTS _____

SPEECH
_____ very clear
_____ pleasant
_____ clear
_____ indistinct

COMMENTS _____

PERSONALITY
_____ magnetic
_____ pleasant
_____ shy
_____ confident
_____ tactless
_____ animated

COMMENTS _____

KNOWLEDGE
_____ clear
_____ understands
_____ uninformed
_____ perceptive
_____ shrewd

COMMENTS _____

INTEREST IN POSITION
_____ exceptional
_____ normal
_____ below average

COMMENTS _____

SUMMARY
_____ superior
_____ above average
_____ average
_____ below average

COMMENTS _____

RECOMMEND EMPLOYMENT
1st choice _____ why _____
2nd choice _____ why _____
3rd choice _____ why _____
4th choice _____ why _____

COMMENTS _____

as **power outage** or **computer crashes**. Remember, it is always better to be *proactive* than *reactive* in business. If you have the **data backed up**, the power outage or crash will mean a short-term headache. If you do not have data backed up, you will never forget the day it happened—or the weeks that followed.

The appointment book should have a column for each technician. The time of the day is an important part of an appointment book and should be boxed off with dark lines for hours and spaced on the 15-minute marks.

Example:
10:00
10:15
10:30
10:45
11:00

When a person calls for an appointment, his or her name should be recorded in pencil when using a paper appointment book so that if the appointment is later canceled, you can easily erase it. When using a computer, you simple delete it. The appropriate time should be on the book for the service, and the type of service should be stated. In most cases, the service will be stated in an abbreviated form. Some of the more standard abbreviations are recorded here. The most important thing is that everyone in your salon and spa should know the meaning of the code you are using.

Service	Abbreviation
Shampoo and style	SS
Service	Abbreviation
Haircut	HC or X
Permanent wave	PERM or PW
Electrolysis	ELEC
Conditioning	C
Hair color	HCL
Body services	BS
Skin care	SC
Lightening	LTN
Manicure	MANI
Pedicure	PEDI

A client's phone number should be taken in case the requested technician becomes ill or cannot make it to work for some reason. Over the time column or next to the name should be a "T" or "R," which will tell if

power outage
A short- or long-term loss of the electric power to an area. Also known as a *power cut, power failure, power loss,* or *blackout.*

computer crash
A condition where a program (either an application or part of the operating system) closes abnormally after encountering an error. Often, the computer program may simply appear to "freeze" or "hang." If this program is a critical part of the operating system kernel, the computer may turn itself off.

data backup
Making copies of data. These additional copies may be used to restore the originals in cases of data loss.

DAY _Thursday_ .... DATE ..... _6/29_ .... 20_01_ .....

OPER.	Cathy (STYLIST)	Jacquie (STYLIST)	Mario (STYLIST)	Lucille (STYLIST)	Joy (MANICURE)	Dorothy (WAXING)	OPER.
8:00	(STYLIST)	(STYLIST)	(STYLIST)	(STYLIST)	(MANICURE)	(WAXING)	8:00
8:15							8:15
8:30							8:30
8:45							8:45
9:00		Carol Gianni		Ellen Adnopaz			9:00
9:15		cut blowdry 555-1874		hair color trim 555-2931			9:15
9:30	Susan White		Telma Brooks		Kerry Moran	Abigail Spiegel	9:30
9:45	shampoo 555-1561		shampoo 555-5668		basic 555-3396	full leg bikini 555-2940	9:45
10:00	cut	Linda Klein	set		Sherri Salem		10:00
10:15		braid 555-4166	Catherine Ross cut blowdry 555-8370	555-9430	tips 555-1647		10:15
10:30	Peggy Neill			Annie Rolland	wraps	Jude Preston	10:30
10:45	hair 555-9853			shampoo cut 555-9430		full leg 555-6324	10:45
11:00	color		Sally McFadden		Lisa Tesar 555-		11:00
11:15			perm 555-2993	Jill Brevda	basic 3010	Pat Keiler 555-0179	11:15
11:30	Barb Matthews	Heidi Blau		cut blowdry 555-8332	Nell Sprock 555-0224	lip/brow	11:30
11:45	cut blowdry 555-7207	hair color 555-8129			french	Sue Axelrod	11:45
12:00				Matt Reagan		full leg bikini 555-4012	12:00
12:15				beard trim 555-1300			12:15
12:30	Kyle Harmon		Laura Deflora		Elisa Klein 555-2817		12:30
12:45	perm 555-1734		perm 555-3276		basic		12:45
1:00	trim	Rich Weller	trim	Ruth Edison	Jim Stein 555-8273	Laura Lowe 555-5107	1:00
1:15		perm 555-8163		perm 555-2705	basic	bikini	1:15
1:30			Claire Sweet	trim	Nancy Goldberg	Denise Carlson 555-4461	1:30
1:45			cut blowdry 555-4278		french 555-1779	arm	1:45
2:00	Allison Nortier			Yolanda Brown		Kendra Miller	2:00
2:15	shampoo cut 555-0127			cut blowdry 555-2576		full leg 555-2704	2:15
2:30	Jennifer Banks	Liz Collito			Linda Douglas		2:30
2:45	hair 555-1320	braid 555-2703			tips 555-1724		2:45
3:00	color		Liz Daley		wraps	Beth Meadows	3:00
3:15			perm 555-2058	Lori Amsdell		lip/brow 555-7190	3:15
3:30			trim	hair 555-7453		bikini	3:30
3:45	Ginny Chamberlan			color	Brenda Turner		3:45
4:00	shampoo cut 555-9673				tips 555-0059	Tracy Brost 555-3712	4:00
4:15					wraps	bikini	4:15
4:30	Mary Porter	Anne Thompson		Elaine Zantos		Jasmine Fine	4:30
4:45	cut blowdry 555-2862	perm 555-1117		cut blowdry 555-2873		lip/brow 555-8623	4:45
5:00		trim	Mary Gallagher	Joe Miranda	Shelli Dills		5:00
5:15			cut blowdry 555-9612	beard trim 555-4800	french 555-4726		5:15
5:30			Pam Jeffries				5:30
5:45	Taryn Liebl		hair 555-8720		Jacquie Flynn		5:45
6:00	perm 555-2878		color		tips 555-8047		6:00
6:15					wraps		6:15

The appointment book should have a column for each *Technician.*

the client is a transit/walk-in or a request customer. Transit/walk-in customers are often exchanged in a salon and spa, while request clients cannot be taken from someone's book without the consent of the client.

When the client enters the salon and spa, a diagonal line is drawn through his or her name, indicating that the client is in the salon and spa. When the client leaves, an "X" is made to indicate that he or she has left the salon and spa and has paid his or her bill (by charging or paying cash).

Most salons and spas using the computer can also now make appointments online. The salon and spa front desk associate usually does this; however, new programs are available to allow the client to book their appointments directly.

APPOINTMENT CARDS

These are cards that confirm a salon and spa appointment. Several things have to be included on these cards. First, they should have the salon and spa's name, address, and telephone number. Next, they should have a space for the time, service, and the technician's name. A small note at the bottom of the card stating, "If an appointment is not canceled at least 24 hours before the time of appointment, a charge will be made," has been an effective means of discouraging customers from not showing up as scheduled. Whether you will actually attempt to collect will depend on your working relationship and respect for the customer. An appointment card is shown below as an example.

Appointment Card

Salon and Spa's Name ....

Address ....

Telephone No. ....

Time .... Service ....

Technician's Name ....

If an appointment is not canceled at least 24 hours before the time of appointment, a charge will be made.

CLIENT RECORD CARDS

Just as you need to educate a client about the way you do business, you need to educate yourself about the way your client operates. The more detailed the information, the more easily you may focus your marketing. Getting more than the name and e-mail address of your client should be a normal part of your process when working with a new client. This information can be stored in your computer data system, or kept manually on cardstock. An example of information below can be formatted to your preference. It can be as detailed or vague as you wish.

Client's Record Card

Client's Name ....

Address ....

Telephone No. ....

E-mail Address ....

Service Received and Date of Service ....

Retail Purchases and Date of Purchase ....

Birthday ....

Occupation ....

Referred By ....

Technician's Name ....

CLIENT EVALUATION CARDS

These should be stored at the front desk associate's desk, but copies filled in by clients should be restricted to the owner/manager. Again, if computerized, this is simply kept on your computer.

Client Evaluation Card

We are in the business to make you feel good about your experience with us!

Making sure you are satisfied and pleased is most important to us. Please help us provide you with the finest quality of service available by answering the questions below. Just give this to the front desk associate when you leave or ask us for a self-addressed, stamped envelope and mail it back at your convenience. We appreciate your response.

Front Desk

Did you find our service to be friendly, professional, and courteous when you:

Called on the telephone?	Yes	No
Asked questions regarding our services?	Yes	No
Scheduled your appointment?	Yes	No
Arrived in the salon?	Yes	No
Paid for your service?	Yes	No

COMMENTS _____

_____

Service

Was the salon staff friendly and helpful?	Yes	No
Was your appointment taken on time?	Yes	No
Were you informed on how to continue a maintenance program for your skin, hair, nails, and other services at home?	Yes	No

Facilities

How would you rate our salon on:

Cleanliness?	Excellent	Good	Fair	Poor
Comfort?	Excellent	Good	Fair	Poor
Lighting?	Excellent	Good	Fair	Poor
Products?	Excellent	Good	Fair	Poor
Music?	Excellent	Good	Fair	Poor
Robes, towels, etc.?	Excellent	Good	Fair	Poor

Reason For Selecting Our Salon:

Friend or associate
Yellow pages
Newspaper
Magazine
Mailing
Gift certificate
Radio
Television
Noticed while driving by
Other _____

COMMENTS _____

_____

What Is Your Overall Impression Of Our Salon?

Excellent   Good   Fair   Poor
How often do you visit a salon? _____

Name _____

Address _____

City _____

State _____ Zip _____

Phone _____

The staff and management want to make sure your visit was most successful. If there are any comments or suggestions you may have, we'd like to know.

_____

_____

Thank you for your time. Your comments make a difference.

■ TECHNICIAN DAILY SALES RECORD SHEETS

This form has several useful features. First, it provides the figures needed to compute a technician's weekly earnings. It carries the technician's name and position, and thus it provides a ready reference.

The chart is divided into several sections relating to each day of the week. If an employee has a day off or is absent from work, a notation can be made for that day. A technician's work is broken down into various activities or services. Note the sample that follows. General work tells of the amount (in dollars and cents) of shampoos, blow-dry services, and haircuts that the technician has performed. You might also incorporate conditioning treatments and other small services in this general term.

Services—that is, hair color, skin care, and makeup—are stated separately in order to track each technician's performance in those categories. As high-ticket items, these can add significantly to a technician's wages and a salon and spa's profitability, but the management must be able to see how much work is being derived from these in order to give assistance where it is needed.

"Other" can include special services—hair weaving, for example—not typical of most salons and spas.

For the sake of simplicity, the salon and spa should pay the same commission on all services. Otherwise, computing payroll can become a bookkeeper's nightmare and can result in increased costs for the salon and spa because more hours must be spent trying to keep the pay record straight.

Additional columns can be added to this sheet as required. These might relate to the time a technician has worked per day and a column for the initials of the technician acknowledging hours worked. When a straight percentage for all work is used to compute a technician's wages, fewer columns will be needed.

■ TECHNICIAN MONTHLY REPORT SHEETS

This form states the technician's name and Social Security number and the totals for the month. These totals should be computed at the end of each week and should be a summary of the technician's daily record sheet, which presents weekly totals. (Note example on page 170.) Shown in this report are:

Technician's Daily Sales Record Sheet

Name _____ Position _____

From Week Beginning _____ To _____

Hours Worked _____

Day	Haircut	Color	Skin Care/Makeup	Waxing	Massage	Mani.	Other	Total	Daily Sales	Total	Retail Sales
Monday											
Tuesday											
Wednesday											
Thursday											
Friday											
Saturday											
Totals											
Last Year's Totals											

Remarks: _____

Technician Monthly Report Sheet

Name .... Social Security no. ....

January 20 .... Hours worked ....

Haircuts ....

Color ....

Skin care/Makeup ....

Waxing ....

Massage ....

Manicure ....

Other ....

Technician's % ....   Technician's wages ....

Total sales ÷ Technician's wages = Salon and spa cost (%) ....

Retail sales ....   Technician's % ....

Total wages of technician ....

Fed. tax $ .... Social Security $ .... State tax $ .... City tax $ ....

Health insurance $ .... Stock purchase $ .... Wages paid $ ....

February 20 .... Hours worked ....

Haircuts ....

Color ....

Skin care/Makeup ....

Waxing ....

Massage ....

Manicure ....

Other ....

Technician's % ....   Technician's wages ....

Total sales ÷ Technician's wages = Salon and spa cost (%) ....

Retail sales ....   Technician's % ....

Total wages of technician ....

Fed. tax $ .... Social Security $ .... State tax $ .... City tax $ ....

Health insurance $ .... Stock purchase $ .... Wages paid $ ....

Note: By placing a ruler running down the page, you can secure all the figures you need to make out your yearly record. Note that all the federal tax, Social Security, state tax, city tax, health insurance, stock purchased, and wages paid amounts are in a straight line.

1. The percentage figures that the salon and spa paid to the employee.
2. The amount that the technician has paid in Social Security, state tax, federal tax, and head tax, and any other deductions that the employee might have made. At the end of the year, a yearly summary should be made for each employee. (Note example on page 170.)

TECHNICIAN YEARLY REPORT FORMS

This form is a compilation of each technician's monthly report sheets. These are kept for 7 years, just in case there is some question about any of the items. You never know when a government official will want a look at your past records. (Note example below on page 172.)

INVENTORY-CONTROL REPORT FORMS

An inventory book, with all supplies, materials, fixtures, working materials, and miscellaneous items, should be kept at the front desk associate's desk or office. This book can be purchased from any office supply store. One book of this type is all that you will need to maintain at a time. A new book should be made each year and should be updated at that time. An example of an inventory control form can be found on page 173.

If inventory-control forms are stored in your computer, the forms can be **zipped** and stored each year also.

zip file
A compressed file that takes up less storage space and therefore can be transferred to other computers quickly.

WANT LIST

A pad of paper or a clipboard to keep a "want list" should be purchased from an office-supply store, and the sheets can be discarded after the supplies have been received. (Note example on page 174.)

REPAIR LIST

A pad of paper or a clipboard to keep a "repair list" should be purchased from an office-supply store. This can be kept in the break room or inventory room. This is primarily for your staff. They sometimes will see things before you will. The sheets can be discarded after the repairs have been completed. (Note example on page 174.)

Technician Yearly Report Form

Year Ending December 20____

Name .... Social Security no. ....

Address .... Phone no. ....

City .... State .... Zip ....

Starting date .... Date of last employment ....

Hours worked ....

Haircut ....

Color ....

Skin care/makeup ....

Waxing ....

Massage ....

Manicure ....

Other ....

Total sales ....

Technician's % ....   Technician's wages ....

Total salon and spa cost..   ÷ 12 (months) = Yearly cost (%) ....

Retail ....   Technician's % ....

Technician's gross yearly wages $ ....

Deductions

Federal tax ....

State tax ....

City tax ....

FICA ....

Health ins. ....

Stock purch ....

Total ....

(−) ....

Total wages paid $ ....

Remarks ....

....

....

		Inventory-Control Report (DATE)		
Code #	**Number of items on hand**	**Inventory description**	**# of items sold January**	**# of items sold to date**
1001	7	XYZ shampoo	49	442
1002	9	XYZ conditioner	25	551
1003	5	XYZ lotion	86	584
1004	9	XYZ clay mask	36	654
1005	6	XYZ body lotion	52	254
1006	5	XYZ sun protector	42	156
1007	10	XYZ polish	69	350
1008	14	XYZ deep conditioner	51	153
1009	5	XYZ hand lotion	45	651
1010	9	XYZ smooth mask	35	453
1011	7	XYZ hand lotion	63	251
1012	6	XYZ SPF 15 protector	25	452
1013	8	XYZ blue shampoo	15	351
1014	4	XYZ blue conditioner	33	213
1015	1	XYZ feet lotion	22	254
1016	2	XYZ clay mask	55	153
1017	3	XYZ body lotion	42	264
1018	5	XYZ sun protector	56	462
1019	4	XYZ shampoo	51	654
1020	6	XYZ conditioner	95	684
1022	5	XYZ clay mask	35	485
1023	0	XYZ body lotion	26	425
1024	3	XYZ body lotion	42	571

Want List

Today's date	....
Item	....
New Item	Yes No
Replaced Item	Yes No

Repair List

Today's date	....
Item	....
Was it discarded?	Yes No
Still in use?	Yes No

▪ DAILY REPORT FORMS FOR SALONS AND SPAS

Daily report forms show the entire business operation of the salon and spa each day. (Note example on next page.) It includes the technicians' intake, retail sales income, and any other money taken in.

The right side of the report shows all the "paid out" items. Bank deposits and money shortages are recorded on this side of the page. The report should contain last year's figures and, if a gross difference appears, a written report should explain this under the heading "Remarks."

Example:

On a certain day, salon and spa sales were 1000.00. Let us say that this indicates that the day was slow. Looking at the technicians' intake, however, we might see that every technician did an increased amount of business, except one. That technician was absent, which explains why the salon and spa was low in business volume that day.

▪ WEEKLY SALON AND SPA REPORT FORMS

Weekly salon and spa report forms are a day-by-day summary of what happened during that week. This information is helpful when it is used to chart a graph that will determine technician vacations and to plan the supply ordering for the next year. (Note example on page 176.)

Daily Report Form (Salon and Spa)

Services Rendered

Technician #1	$ ....
Technician #2	$ ....
Technician #3	$ ....
Technician #4	$ ....
Total services rendered	$ ....

Retail Sales

Shampoo	$ ....
Conditioner	$ ....
Styling aids	$ ....
	$ ....
Specials	$ ....
	$ ....
Total retail sales	$ ....
Misc. sales	$ ....
	$ ....
Total misc. sales	$ ....
Vending machine	$ ....
Total business of the day	$ ....

Bank statement

Cash	$ ....
Checks	$ ....
Coins	$ ....
Total deposit	$ ....
Charges	1. $ ....
	2. $ ....
Total charges	$ ....

Cash Paid Out

1. ....
2. ....
3. ....
4. Refunds

    A. ....

    B. ....

    Reasons: ....

    ....

Total cash paid out $ ....

Bills

Received	Paid	Held
1.	....	....
2.	....	....
3.	....	....

Cash Report

Total business		$ ....
Currency	(+)	$ ....
Coins	(+)	$ ....
Checks	(+)	$ ....
Total cash		$ ....
+ Total charges		$ ....
Total		$ ....
− Cash to start		$ ....
Total business		$ ....
Long	Short	
Last year $..........	This year $	
Remarks: ....
....

Weekly Salon and Spa Report Form

Services Rendered by Technicians

Monday ....

Tuesday ....

Wednesday ....

Thursday ....

Friday ....

Saturday ....

Total services $ ....

Retail Sales

Monday ....

Tuesday ....

Wednesday ....

Thursday ....

Friday ....

Saturday ....

Total retail sales $ ....

Misc. and Vending Machine Sales

Monday ....

Tuesday ....

Wednesday ....

Thursday ....

Friday ....

Saturday ....

Total misc. and
vending machine $ ....

Total gross sales
for week $ ....

Balance $ ....

Cash Paid Out

Monday ....

Tuesday ....

Wednesday ....

Thursday ....

Friday ....

Saturday ....

Total cash paid out $ ....

Bills

	Received	Paid	Held
Monday		....	....
Tuesday		....	....
Wednesday		....	....
Thursday		....	....
Friday		....	....
Saturday		....	....
Total bills received	$		

Bank Deposits

Monday ....

Tuesday ....

Wednesday ....

Thursday ....

Friday ....

Saturday ....

Total bank deposits
for week $ ....

Total cash paid out $ ....

Total bills paid $ ....

Total $ ....

Balance $ ....

▪ MONTHLY SALON AND SPA REPORT FORMS

Monthly salon and spa report forms provide a summary of weekly operations. They are used to establish bonus figures for each employee when such compensation is involved. It is also a complete summary of what happened in your salon and spa that month. From this, you can see if you made a profit for the month or if a special promotional activity has helped your sales over the last year. In evaluating monthly figures, be sure that you are looking at base figures. If the price you charge for a shampoo and set has gone up during the year, the base figure could be different. (Note example on page 178.)

Example:
Comparing figures shows that the salon and spa made an increase in sales this year of 8 percent. On the surface this looks good. If, however, you raised prices 12 percent over the past year, you are actually running behind last year in business volume.

▪ YEARLY REPORTS ON SALON AND SPA ACTIVITIES

After you have the 12 monthly salon and spa report forms completed, you will have little trouble figuring **taxes**, wages, **profits**, and cost. From this information, you should compile and write a yearly report. (Note example on page 179.) In this report, you should state your profit, what you lost money on, amounts you paid out in all areas, and, most important, what you intend to do in the future. This is important because it establishes, in writing, a direction for your salon and spa. Furthermore, if you should sell the salon and spa, die, or become unable to run the salon and spa, the person who takes your place knows where you have been and where you are heading. Your accountant may also find it helpful when counseling you on finance.

tax
The imposition of a financial charge or other levy upon a taxpayer (an individual or legal entity) by a state or the functional equivalent of a state such that failure to pay is punishable by law.

profit
The positive financial gain, after all expenses have been subtracted, from an investment or business operation.

▪ TECHNICIAN SERVICE SHEETS

These usually take the form of printed tickets. They consist of the technician's name, the customer's name, the service rendered, the date, and the cost of the service. The customer will regard this as his or her bill and will pay the total amount at the front desk associate's

Monthly Salon and Spa Report Form

Services Rendered by Technicians

Week 1 ....

Week 2 ....

Week 3 ....

Week 4 ....

Week 5 ....

Total monthly services $ ....

Retail Sales

Week 1 ....

Week 2 ....

Week 3 ....

Week 4 ....

Week 5 ....

Total monthly retail sales $ ....

Misc. and Vending Machine Sales

Week 1 ....

Week 2 ....

Week 3 ....

Week 4 ....

Week 5 ....

Total misc. and vending
machine sales $ ....

Total sales $ ....

Balance $ ....

Total Cash Paid Out

Week 1 ....

Week 2 ....

Week 3 ....

Week 4 ....

Week 5 ....

Total cash paid out $ ....

Bills

Received	Paid	Held
Week 1	....	....
Week 2	....	....
Week 3	....	....
Week 4	....	....
Week 5	....	....
Total bills recevied	$	$ ....

Bank Deposits

Week 1 ....

Week 2 ....

Week 3 ....

Week 4 ....

Week 5 ....

Total monthly deposits $ ....

Total cash paid out $ ....

Total bills received $ ....

Total bills paid $ ....

Bills received but
not paid $ ....

Yearly Report on Salon and Spa Activities

Year Ending December 20.......

	Gross Technicians' Sales	Gross Retail Sales	Misc. and Vending Machines	Special Sales
January				
February				
March				
April				
May				
June				
July				
August				
September				
October				
November				
December				
Total				

Gross sales from technicians' personal supplies $ ....

Other sales

1. ....

2. ....

3. .... $ ....

Gross income from 20.......... $ ....

desk. The tally remains the property of the salon and spa, regardless of how the customer pays the bill. Keep tally sheets, sales tickets, and/or the computer records of these for the time prescribed by law—seven years— as they are important tax records of technicians' services rendered and appointments kept. If there is a question about the amount of business done on a given day by a technician, all that is needed to answer the question is to add the tallies of that particular technician. Tickets

Expenses

	Gross Technicians' Wages	Supplies	Laundry Expense	Retail Items
January				
February				
March				
April				
May				
June				
July				
August				
September				
October				
November				
December				
Total				

	Misc. Costs	Federal Tax	State Tax	Local Tax	FICA	Licenses
January						
February						
March						
April						
May						
June						
July						
August						
September						
October						
November						
December						
Total						

Expenses (Cont.)
Additional Costs

January $ ....

....

....

....

February $ ....

....

....

....

March $ ....

....

....

....

April $ ....

....

....

....

May $ ....

....

....

....

June $ ....

....

....

....

July $ ....

....

....

....

August $ ....

....

....

....

Expenses (Cont.)
Additional Costs (Cont.)

September $ ....

....

....

....

October $ ....

....

....

November $ ....

....

....

December $ ....

....

....

....

	Total additional cost	$	

Total technicians' wages	$	Total federal tax	$ ....
Total supply cost	$	Total state tax	$ ....
Total laundry expense	$	Total FICA	$ ....
Total retail items cost	$	Total licenses	$ ....
Total additional cost	$	Total misc. cost	$ ....
Total yearly expenses	$		
Gross income for 20_____	$		
Yearly expenses (−)	$		
Gross profit	$		

Cost of money
    (interest on principal from bank mortgage) $ ....

Money paid on principal $ ....

Total $ ....

Net profit (gross profit − money cost and principal payment) $ ....

Expenses (Cont.)
Additional Costs
(Cont.)

Remarks:

....

....

....

....

Future Technician Plans:

....

....

....

....

---

should be numbered so that extra tickets cannot be added or sub-tracted. If your salon and spa accepts credit cards, the client will receive one copy. The others are for your own records and to send to the credit-card company for their own records and billing purposes.

■ BANK DEPOSIT RECORD BOOK

This is a book in which all deposits are recorded by the bank. It is given to the salon and spa by the bank, and each day, as deposits are made, they are recorded. The deposit book contains the account number, the date of transaction, and the initials of the teller who takes the deposit. This book then becomes a ready reference for the amount you

---

An example:
Account Number 70-2345

Date	Amount	Teller
4-1-20____	$250.00	J. W.
4-2-20____	$323.00	B. V.
4-3-20____	$274.25	J. R.

have in the bank. The amount of each deposit should be entered immediately in the computer accounting files in order to avoid mistakes. If you use an automatic teller machine, be sure to keep the record of the transaction until the deposit is recorded on your next statement.

■ BANK DEPOSIT RECEIPTS

Deposit receipts are receipts for the money you have deposited at the bank. They should show the same amount that the salon and spa grossed the day before (the charges). These receipts should be stapled to the daily salon and spa report and filed away with it.

■ CHECKBOOK

This book of checks is for salon and spa use only. Any check written on this account should be for a business expense. Personal checks written on business accounts cause tax problems and pave the way to a bankrupt salon and spa. The checkbook comes in several forms, with several types of information stubs. Your banker will help you select the proper type for your particular business.

■ EMPLOYEES' TIP REPORT FORMS

Tip reporting form can be obtained by writing your local Internal Revenue Service (IRS) office. These forms are given to all employees. Employees are required to state the amount of **tips** over a specified figure and return the form to you. You are required to withhold taxes on that amount from their regular salary checks. This is a safeguard for the technicians so that they will not end the year owing the government additional income tax.

Within the last year, a new item has surfaced. When a client pays by a credit card and adds a "tip" for the stylist, the salon and spa gives the tip to the stylist. However, the salon and spa deducts the cost of the credit card transaction, the taxes due (local, state, and federal governments), and **FICA**. The *net* amount is then added to the employee's wages and is paid at the same time as regular services rendered.

---

tip report form

A form that can be obtained by writing the local Internal Revenue Service (IRS) office. These forms are given to all employees, who are required to declare the amount of tips over a specified figure and return the form to the salon and spa owner/manager.

tip

A compensation arrangement in which the client, to ensure prompt/proper service, gives a certain amount over and above the stated price of a service to the technician who performed the service. Cosmetologists often make a considerable portion of their income from client tips.

FICA

Payroll taxes for Social Security benefits collected under the authority of the Federal Insurance Contributions Act, or FICA.

There is also the option to be a **nontipping** establishment. This is a trend we have seen in the industry strongly for the last 10 years. You may find this is a point of difference for your new business also.

nontipping
A decision not to accept tips as a form of payment.

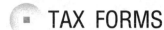

TAX FORMS

Forms for collecting and remitting tax money can be obtained free from any IRS office. In some cases, you will have three or more forms to fill out and send: one for the federal government, one for the state government, one for city head tax, and/or income tax. State sales tax, federal sales tax, and taxes on vending machines may all have to be remitted. Forms for each of these should accompany your salon and spa's tax payment check.

Chapter 13 Summary

- The forms you use will determine whether you have on hand the information you will need to run your business.

- One of the most important records kept in the salon and spa is the appointment book, whether it is stored in a paper book, or on the computer system. This should contain information about your clients, how often they come in, and what services they use.

- Always backing up electronic files will save you from unneeded stress.

Review Questions

1. What can you do to be proactive instead of reactive when managing your computer system?

2. What are two differences between a walk-in and a request client?

3. What is the difference between a "client record card" and a "client evaluation card"? Discuss what each contains and how they are used.

4. How might a salon and spa owner use a weekly salon and spa report form?

5. What information is found on a technician's service sheet? How can it be used to help the technician?

[1]If an accountant is doing your bookkeeping, he or she will have these forms and all related information available in his or her office. A good accountant can save the salon and spa time, effort, energy, and money because of his or her knowledge of the tax structure and tax requirements.

Answers to Review Questions

Chapter 1

1. Answers will vary. Potential answers may include, but are not limited to:
   a. Salons used to be much smaller operations, with one to four employees.
   b. Typically, women used to go to beauty salons and men to barbers.
   c. The services offered at salons and spas have expanded to include additional services such as massage therapy, skin care, manicure/pedicure, and other related services.

2. Answers will vary. Potential answers may include, but are not limited to:
   a. Department store/fitness center salons and spas often contract with a nationwide chain of salons.
   b. Department store/fitness center salons and spas often supply an audit facility and accounting system.
   c. Hotel salons and spas are sometimes able to use a system that allows hotel guests to charge spa services to their hotel tab.
   d. Hotel salons and spas may offset the lack of shopping by expanding their service menu to include full-body massage, makeup, hair removal, body wraps, Botox injections, manicures, acrylic nails, pedicures, false eyelashes, permanent makeup, or other services.

3. Answers will vary. Potential answers may include, but are not limited to:
   Similarities:
   a. In both cases, the law does not distinguish between the business and its owners.
   b. In both cases, decisions made to benefit the salon and spa must follow all current state and federal laws and regulations
   c. Whether the salon and spa is shared by multiple owners or a sole proprietor, liability for what happens in the salon and spa still rests on the individual(s) who have legal ownership of the salon.
   Differences:
   a. Sole proprietorships are owned by one person; partnerships are owned by two or more people.
   b. Sole proprietors own all assets of the business; partners share the assets of the business.
   c. Sole proprietors receive all of the profits generated by the business; partners share the profits generated by the business.

4. Answers will vary. Potential answers may include, but are not limited to:
   a. Maintain good communication and healthy relationships with the stylists working around you.
   b. Always consider how your actions may impact your reputation and your business.

c. Stay up-to-date regarding state and federal laws.

5. The most common way people will find you online is by searching for your salon and spa name.

Chapter 2

1. Leasing may be a better option than paying cash if you do not have any money to put down. However, paying cash up front reduces your expenses each month.

2. Answers will vary. Potential answers may include, but are not limited to:

   a. The bank may require collateral.

   b. The bank may require good credit.

   c. The bank may require detailed financial reporting, including tax records and proposed planning for requested financing.

   d. The approval process may take too long for your business needs.

3. With a secured loan, lenders will take a security interest in your property and have the right to seize your collateral if payments are not received. With an unsecured loan, the lender loans money based solely on the credit of the borrower. It is not secured with collateral.

4. Private lenders can receive a higher interest rate than they would get from an investment or if they just put their money in the bank.

5. Beauty-supply distributors can guarantee the integrity of the equipment, and they can loan you equipment if yours fails.

Chapter 3

1. The salon and spa would need to produce $16.50 per hour.

   $78,000 (goal)/52 (weeks in a year) = $1,500 per week

$1,500 (weekly goal)/100 (hours per week) = $15 per hour

Add a 10% profit margin ($1.50) = $15.00 + $1.50 = $16.50

2. The "list" price of a product is the price on a unit of merchandise where the unit represents several items. Cost is lowered because there is only one order, one delivery, and no odd units of merchandise are left. The "deal" price also involves purchasing multiple units, but you must purchase the merchandise during a given period. If you purchase a certain amount, you will get an additional amount free.

3. Answers will vary. Potential answers may include, but are not limited to:

   a. Manage your inventory carefully. Do not have more than a two-weeks' supply on hand, but do not run out, either.

   b. Train and encourage staff to sell products. Promotions should support sales, and staff should be assertive about selling product.

   c. Practice good buying habits. Take advantage of promotions, but do not buy product that you cannot sell.

4. Wages must be low enough so a salon and spa can make a reasonable profit. Wages must also be high enough to attract and maintain good technicians.

Chapter 4

1. Answers will vary. Potential answers may include, but are not limited to:

   a. If the building site contains asbestos, it will have to be removed at considerable expense.

   b. The building may have problems with the electrical wiring or water damage.

   c. The building may have structural damage caused by termites or other vermin.

2. Without a sales tax license, you cannot sell any retail in your salon and spa.

3. Answers will vary. Potential answers may include, but are not limited to:
   a. Gas and electric: Supply name, address, name/nature of your business, three credit references, and possibly a deposit.
   b. Telephone: Supply a deposit and pay separate fee to have the phone installed.
   c. Trash removal: Supply name, address, name of your business and when service should start. Verify if you need to supply your own trash container.
   d. Local police and fire department: Indicate who owns the salon and spa, where they can be reached, the salon and spa hours, and staff contact information (in case you cannot be reached).

4. Answers will vary. Potential answers may include, but are not limited to:
   a. Are there any cancellation clauses?
   b. Will my rate increase due to claims?
   c. Is cancellation automatic after a number of claims have been made during a policy year?
   d. Are claims honored for out-of-court as well as in-court settlements?
   e. How much money will I receive during the time that settlement cases or court deliberations keep me away from the salon and spa?
   f. Who will pay the costs of witnesses and other related expenses?

5. Liability insurance protects you in situations where someone has an accident on your property. Malpractice insurance protects the salon and spa and technicians in situations where neglect or misuse of a product has resulted in injury while a service was rendered.

Chapter 5

1. a. Note all damaged or missing items before moving in and have the manager sign the list.

   b. Take a picture before you move in and after you move out, and include them with your list.

2. Construction in or near your salon and spa may cost you a significant portion of your business through decreased regular clientele, walk-in traffic, and even staff. The clause ensures that you will receive space that is the same size or larger after any remodeling. A salon and spa owner should request a lower rent during the remodel period and possibly longer while business returns to normal.

3. A single-business clause states that your salon and spa is the only one in the leasing area. This prevents a cut-rate salon and spa or beauty school from opening within a certain distance of your salon and spa. An exclusive clause is based on services and would prevent your landlord from allowing direct competitors like nail or massage businesses from opening within a certain distance of your salon.

4. Answers will vary. Potential answers may include, but are not limited to:
   a. Is the location convenient to the clientele you wish to serve?
   b. What are the costs per square foot of other competitive locations?
   c. What are the zoning restrictions, traffic counts, and visibility of the space?
   d. What are the demographics of the people who work, shop, or live in the area?

Chapter 6

1. Answers will vary. Potential answers may include, but are not limited to:
   a. Clean hair spray, dust, and fingerprints off the windows regularly to ensure that the glass remains clear.
   b. Display one item clearly rather than several items competing with each other.

c. Change displays often and keep up with trends.

d. Use words like *Free, Complimentary, Gift,* and so forth to entice walk-ins.

2. Retail racks should be accessible to clients near the front desk associate, but not behind the front desk associate. Customers should be able to pick up, touch, smell, and read the packaging on products. Products should be near the front desk associate so that he or she can offer advice and answer any questions.

3. Fluorescent tube lights produce the most light and are the most inexpensive to operate; the new tubes give almost perfect reproduction of sunlight. Chandeliers are used for their beauty and to give light.

4. Answers will vary. Potential answers may include, but are not limited to:

a. Consider your clientele when selecting your magazines. The magazines should reflect their interests.

b. You should have about three magazines per technician working in your salon.

c. Magazines should be changed frequently and should be removed as soon as they are damaged or outdated.

d. Magazines should never be left on chairs or on the floor. They should be in a magazine rack or on a table.

e. Recycle the magazines and build your business by donating the old and outdated copies to rest homes, senior centers, and hospitals.

5. Answers will vary. Potential answers may include, but are not limited to:

a. The entire service can be done at a wet station. This saves time compared to a dry station, where a client would have to be moved to have his or her hair shampooed.

b. The client never has to be moved from a wet station during a service, unlike a dry station, which is particularly important if your client has any mobility issues.

c. Each stylist is responsible for his or her station, its cleanliness, and how well it is stocked. There is no need to share stations, like when using a dry station.

d. If the salon and spa does not have to share a shampoo station, as stylists would if everyone had dry stations, a client's shampoo will never interfere with another client's service.

Chapter 7

1. The "original composition" of the salon and spa refers to how the salon was built. The walls, floors, and ceiling in good repair project a desirable image for the salon. Well-designed plumbing and electrical connections, brushes, combs, manicuring equipment, towels, and robes are all necessary components for a successful service.

2. a. Care for the physical and psychological needs of the salon.

b. Provide guidance for each employee and help them succeed.

c. Retain decision-making power, but let the staff have a voice and offer advice on how they think you should go forward.

d. Invest in yourself! Attend management trainings.

3. Answers will vary. Potential answers may include, but are not limited to:

a. Computer systems: A computer system is important to a salon and spa business because it is used to perform many important functions such as managing payroll, inventory, and bank deposits. To maximize use, ensure that you choose the correct program for your salon and have multiple people trained on the system to ensure that you always have someone in the salon who is familiar with the system.

b. Bookkeeping system: A bookkeeping system is important to a salon and spa business because it helps ensure that employees are paid correctly and on time. This helps maintain a positive morale in the salon and can increase staff retention.

4. Answers will vary. Potential answers may include, but are not limited to:

   a. Keep an up-to-date inventory on hand at all times.

   b. Make a "want list" and have it handy.

   c. Always place and store merchandise wisely and safely.

   d. Take time with your supply representative when placing your order.

5. Answers will vary. Potential answers may include, but are not limited to:

   a. Keep your supplies arranged in an orderly fashion.

   b. When new merchandise comes into the salon and spa, be sure that the old merchandise is brought to the front to be used first.

   c. Ensure that no supply shelf is more than 1 foot deep.

   d. Store cosmetics away from heaters and dryers to avoid spoiling.

   e. Keep products away from the sink unless needed for shampooing.

Chapter 8

1. A slogan can be used externally to advertise or internally as part of a mission statement. Included in the slogan should be the key attributes of your business that set you apart from the competition.

2. Answers will vary. Potential answers may include, but are not limited to:

   a. Web site: Share basic information as well as promotions with current and future customers.

   b. E-mail: A free way to distribute promotions to your existing customers.

   c. Social-networking sites: Free way to promote your business and talk about what services you provide.

   d. Search engines: Free exposure through the regular results of the search engine.

3. Answers will vary. Potential answers may include, but are not limited to:

   a. The marketing will reach the people most likely to come to your salon, since 90 percent of salon clients typically live or work within a 5-mile radius of the salon.

   b. Direct mail can entice first-time clients with your services, products, and promotions.

   c. Direct mail can keep your present clients informed of your services, products, and promotions.

4. Answers will vary. Potential answers may include, but are not limited to:

   a. Always make sure your clients look their best when they leave your salon and have the products they need to maintain their look between visits.

   b. Give your clients your complete attention while they are in your salon chair.

   c. Simply ask for a referral.

   d. Hand out your business cards.

   e. Tell people you meet what you do and where your salon is.

5. Answers will vary. Potential answers may include, but are not limited to:

   a. How many calls came from the ad? This can tell you how many people were interested enough by your advertisement to request more information.

   b. How many appointments were booked? What services were rendered and did they prebook for a returning service? These questions can tell you if your advertisement is attracting the people who are a fit for your salon.

   c. Track how many new customers responded. This can tell you if you are expanding your client base through the advertisement.

   d. Compare what you spent on the promotion to what you earned. Did you make more money than you spent? (Remember to consider the new customers that you attracted who prebooked for another appointment.)

e. What are other businesses in the area doing to advertise? You may discover new ideas for your salon or a local business with which you can pair up to share client lists and mailing costs.

Chapter 9

1. Gross sales are the total amount of money taken in by the salon and spa during the year, whereas real profit is a term used to describe the amount of money left after all the bills have been paid.
2. Have a guest or stylist speak to motivate the salon and spa. Require attendance and cover important topics such as human relations, communication, salesmanship, new products, and service techniques and sales results.
3. The client will share patterns with the technician that will help the technician choose the best services. This will lead to customer satisfaction.
4. a. Explain the importance of rebooking! It ensures that the stylist will be available when the client is ready to return to the salon. Offer to provide a reminder call the day before the appointment.
   b. If the client is still not interested in rebooking, the front desk associate/technician should give the client the technician's business card.
5. Answers will vary. Potential answers may include, but are not limited to:
   a. Be proactive instead of reactive when planning a promotion.
   b. Establish your customers' needs before choosing a promotion.
   c. If you are moving into selling a new kind of merchandise (like jewelry or clothing)

start small so that you do not risk too much of your capital.
   d. Be consistent in your template each year. Save your promotions from year to year on a CD or flash drive.
   e. Create bins for monthly promotions.
   f. Consider what would motivate the staff to support the promotion.

Chapter 10

1. It may be true that the client does not want to change to a trendy look, but the technician can never really know unless he or she asks. It is the technician's responsibility to help his or her clients stay up to date, and this includes checking in with clients, even if there is no reason to think they are interested in a change.
2. Consumers in salons and spas demand certain services and, as a result, employers look to schools for the related skills in their graduates. A partnership helps schools understand what is needed in the current salon and spa environment and helps salons and spas get the skills they are looking for in graduates.
3. Answers will vary. Potential answers may include, but are not limited to, the following. A cosmetology instructor can tell an employer about a stylist's:
   a. Personality. What is his or her typical disposition?
   b. Customer service skills. Did the stylist develop a clientele at the school? How did he or she treat a customer?
   c. Willingness to cooperate. Does he or she work well with others?
   d. Attitude. What is his or her outlook on work?
   e. Technical skills. What are his or her greatest strengths? Weaknesses?
   f. Telephone approach. Is he or she friendly and professional on the phone?

4. Answers will vary. Potential answers may include, but are not limited to:
   a. Visit the schools—Helps students view you as an industry expert, not just someone who comes to the school when needing to hire.
   b. Teach specialty classes at the school—What technique do you love? Give back to the community by sharing the passion that you have with students.
   c. Participate in job fairs—Set up a table; give away fun, inexpensive items; and be available to answer questions.
   d. Offer tours of your salon and spa—Allow students to experience your salon environment.
   e. Leave information about your salon at the school—Provide people with materials they can review when they have free time.
   f. Offer student and teacher discounts—Give them a fun incentive to come in.

Chapter 11

1. All applicants have to be treated the same and scored on the same criteria.
2. First, all people must be provided equal treatment under the law. Second, it is reasonable to assume that the male employee may be needed to provide assistance to the mother and child.
3. A reasonable accommodation may include the addition of a ramp for a wheelchair or the removal of a decorative barrier. An excessive accommodation would include anything that would cost the organization more money than the employee would generate.
4. Employers must pay employees the federal minimum wage and overtime pay to nonexempt employees.
5. Answers will vary. Potential answers may include, but are not limited to:

Strengths:
1. An employment contract gives the business a chance to recoup the cost of hiring a new employee.
2. The employee usually agrees not to work within a certain distance of the salon after separation from the organization.
3. Some court cases have favored the employer.

Weaknesses:
1. Circumstances may not allow you to enforce the contract. For example, being in a small town with a small number of salons in which technicians can work could make an agreement not to work within a certain distance of the salon after separation an unreasonable request.
2. Some court cases have favored the employee.

Chapter 12

1. Answers will vary. Potential answers may include, but are not limited to:
   a. In the newspaper, the heading on the advertisement will help people easily notice your advertisement.
   b. In the newspaper, you will place your advertisement under "Help Wanted, Professional" and are likely to reach the best local candidates.
   c. Marketing on the Web will give you the largest pool of candidates since your advertisement can be accessed from anywhere in the world.
   d. Your Web advertisement can be found when people go to the site that you posted it or through a search engine.
   e. You will not be charged per letter in a Web advertisement (unlike a newspaper advertisement) so you can be more detailed in your job description.

2. Answers will vary. Potential answers may include, but are not limited to:

   a. Marketing—You may have to spend money to find a replacement.

   b. Loss of clientele—People coming to your salon and spa may follow the technician to his or her new salon and spa.

   c. Sales promotion—Money, time, and effort will be needed to get a new stylist up to speed.

   d. Additional salaries—Other people may need to work additional hours to cover for the separated employee.

3. In a commission salon and spa, the technician is paid based on the services that he or she generates. This allows the maximum amount of control over their earnings. Hourly salons and spas also often have incentive programs, but they are not tied as closely to daily technical production.

4. A salon and spa duty list helps clarify expectations for every employee. Motivate stylists to keep the salon and spa clean by talking to them about why cleanliness is important and how it can improve their clients' experiences.

5. Answers will vary. Potential answers may include, but are not limited to:

   a. Your dress policy should reflect the image of the salon and spa. This will attract desirable employees and clients.

   b. Hair should be styled and should be a result of work done in that salon and spa, not a competitor's salon and spa. Items sold in the salon and spa such as wigs, clips, and so forth should be worn as much as possible. Technicians can be the greatest advertisement you have if everyone remembers to give consideration to their image every day.

   c. Tattoos and piercings should be covered if they are inappropriate. Technicians could inadvertently decrease their own business potential.

   d. Shoes should be clean and neat. It is important to have a clean and neat image, and appropriate shoes are also a potential safety and a licensing issue.

   e. Female stylists should wear makeup every day, and male stylists should shave (or trim their facial hair) every day. Technicians are in the beauty industry and appearance is important.

Chapter 13

1. Back up the computer system at the end of every day. Print out the appointments for the next day the night before. If the computer crashes, only the recent data will be affected.

2. a. A walk-in client requests a service from someone in the salon and spa. A request client asks for a service from a specific technician.

   b. A walk-in client may be moved from one technician to another easily, but a request client cannot be moved without the client's consent.

3. A client's record card contains information *about* the client, such as name, contact information, service preferences, and birth date. It is used by the stylist to provide a better, more customized service experience. A client evaluation card is *filled out by* the client and asks questions about the client's experience in the salon and spa. It is used to make improvements to the salon and spa and to make the salon and spa more appealing.

4. The weekly salon and spa report form can be used to plan vacations for the next year and to order supplies more accurately based on business flow.

5. The technician service sheet has the technician's name, the customer's name, the service rendered, the date, and the cost of the service. The technician needs them specifically for tax purposes, and they are a valuable part of accurate record-keeping in general.

Glossary

accidental deletion The unintended removal of client information, files, or documents.

accountant A practitioner of accountancy, who is licensed to practice the measurement, disclosure, or provision of assurance about financial statistics and information.

additional salary All income given over and above regular salary.

administrative staff Persons employed by the business owner who are hired to conduct daily business operations, such as a manager or front desk associate.

assistant Within the beauty industry, a person who aids and supports beauty technicians; a technician in training.

bankruptcy When an individual or company has been declared, by law, to be unable to pay its debts to creditors or individuals.

bookkeeper A person who records the financial transactions of a person or business, including sales, purchases, income, and payments.

bookkeeping system The process that a bookkeeper uses to record the financial trans-actions of an individual or business.

booth rental System in which a renter leases space, or a "booth," within a salon and spa. The renter then uses the space to operate his or her own business for personal financial benefit, rather than for the success of the overall salon and spa.

branding A sign, name, or symbol used to identify a business, service, or specific product.

capital gain Profit that results from selling stocks, bonds, or real estate at a price that exceeds the purchase price. The result is a financial gain for the investor.

capital investment Money that is invested in the business with the expectation of income, and recovered through earnings generated by the business over several years.

CEU credit Continuing-education classes to keep a professional license.

collateral Security pledged for the payment of a loan.

commission Revenue derived from services provided, paid to the technician performing those services.

computer crash A condition where a program (either an application or part of the operating system) closes abnormally after encountering an error. Often, the computer program may simply appear to "freeze" or "hang." If this program is a critical part of the operating system kernel, the computer may turn itself off.

computer system A programmable machine that receives input, stores and manipulates data/information, and provides output in a useful format.

corporation An institution that is granted a charter recognizing it as a separate legal entity having its own privileges, and liabilities distinct from those of its members.

cosmetology The study and application of beauty treatment. Branches of specialty including hairstyling, skin care, cosmetics, and manicures/pedicures.

cost of goods sold The inventory costs of those goods the business has sold during a particular period of time.

creditworthiness A creditor's measure of an individual's or company's ability to meet debt obligations.

customer service A series of activities created to improve the level of customer satisfaction. "Exceed customer expectation."

customer Also known as a *client, guest,* or *purchaser*; a current or potential buyer or user of the products and services provided by the business.

customer's goodwill The value of intangible assets such as a strong brand name, good customer relations, and good employee relations.

cyber platform An Internet environment used as platforms for ad delivery.

data backup Making copies of data. These additional copies may be used to restore the original in the case of data loss.

demographics The profiles of characteristics of a population used in government, marketing, or opinion research.

department store/fitness center salon and spa A salon and spa that usually operates in a leased-space area. Major department stores and fitness centers usually contract with a nationwide chain of salons and spas, and their operations can vary from a small salon and spa to a multiunit salon and spa of 30 to 60 technicians.

depreciation A decline in value of assets.

domain name An identification label that defines a realm of administrative autonomy, authority, or control on the Internet.

due diligence An investigation of a business or person prior to signing a contract, most commonly applied to voluntary investigations. However, can also be a legal obligation.

economic condition A state at a particular time; "a condition (or state) of disrepair"; "the condition of finances.

electronic media Media that use electronic or electromechanical energy for the end user to access the content.

e-mail address An e-mail mailbox to which e-mail messages may be received and from which e-mail messages may be delivered.

e-mail marketing The use of e-mail as a means of communicating commercial or fund-raising messages to bring customers to the business and generate sales.

employee A person who is hired to provide services to a company on a regular basis in exchange for compensation and who does not provide these services as part of an independent business.

employee discount Often used as incentive to work for a company, a discount on services or a percentage off products.

employee-owned corporation A business arrangement in which employees own stock in the company, which they purchase when the company is formed or which they earn as part of their compensation over the years.

employment contract A traditional written agreement that is signed and agreed to by employer and employee.

entrepreneur A person who has possession of a new enterprise, venture, or idea and assumes significant accountability for the inherent risks and the outcome.

equity The value of an ownership interest in property, including shareholders' equity in a business.

esthetician Also called *skin care therapist*; a technician who works at salons, day spas, and medispas; is trained in the cosmetic treatment of the skin; performs various cosmetic procedures including facials, body treatments, and waxing; and usually offers a variety of specialty spa treatments.

FICA Payroll taxes for Social Security benefits collected under the authority of the Federal Insurance Contributions Act, or FICA.

financing Saving money and, often, lending money. How money is spent and budgeted within the business.

fixed loan A loan in which the interest rate is guaranteed not to change for a specified period.

flex dollars A term used to assign values to employees benefits.

franchise A business licensed to sell and market a parent company's goods and services, operating under the same name, and using the parent company's successful business model.

freestanding salon and spa A salon and spa whose structure is not attached to another structure.

front desk associate An information clerk who is responsible for dealing with clients and who has a significant impact on the success of an organization.

general partnership A business arrangement in which partners divide responsibility for management and liability, as well as the shares of profit or loss, according to their internal agreement. Equal shares are assumed unless there is a written agreement that states differently.

gross income An individual's or business's total income before taking taxes or deductions.

gross sales The total amount of money taken in by the salon and spa during the year; overall sales, before deducting operating expenses, cost of goods sold, payment of taxes, or any other expenses.

hard copy A physical object, permanent reproduction, or copy. Any media suitable for direct use by a person to view displayed or transmitted data.

hardware An object that is tangible, such as disks, disk drives, display screens, keyboards, printers, boards, and chips.

hotel salon and spa A salon and spa that has been expanded into a day spa due to the hotel/resort's distance from other retail outlets. Services range from hair services to full-body massage, makeup, hair removal, body wraps, Botox injections, manicure, acrylic nails, pedicures, false eyelashes, permanent makeup, and a host of other services.

hourly + bonuses A compensation arrangement in which, in addition to an hourly wage, a percentage of the money made from the provision of services is given back to the cosmetologist as income when certain predetermined goals are obtained.

hourly + salary A compensation arrangement in which, in addition to an hourly wage, a periodic payment is given to the cosmetologist as income.

IRS Internal Revenue Service.

Internet A global system of interconnected computer networks that serve billions of users worldwide.

Internet access The means by which users connect to the Internet.

Internet ad Online advertising, a form of promotion that uses the World Wide Web for the express purpose of delivering marketing messages to attract customers.

inventory system The process to keep track of objects or materials for the business. Many inventory-control systems rely upon barcodes or RFID tags.

joint venture A legal entity formed between two or more parties to undertake an economic activity together, like a general partnership but clearly for a limited period of time or a single project.

landlord The owner of lands, buildings, property, and so forth that are rented or leased to an individual or business, called the *tenant.*

lawsuit A civil action brought before a court of law in which the plaintiff claims to have received damages from a defendant's actions and is now seeking a legal or equitable remedy.

lease agreement A contract by which the landlord (or lessor) gives the tenant (or lessee) the use and possession of lands, buildings, property, and so forth, for a specified time and in return for fixed payments.

leased-space and booth-rental The latest ownership model in which the owner contracts for a given area of space and subdivides the space into several rooms or studios, much like a doctor's office, and each room is rented to a practitioner for a service.

license Means "to give permission"; a license may be issued by authorities, allowing an activity that would otherwise be forbidden.

limited liability company (LLC) A business arrangement that provides the limited-liability features of a corporation and the tax efficiencies and operational flexibility of a partnership.

logo A graphic mark or emblem to aid and promote instant public recognition. Logos are either purely graphic (symbols/icons) or composed of the name of the organization.

mall/shopping center salon and spa A salon and spa located within a mall/shopper center that may rely on the convenience of a collection of independent retail stores and services. Normally they are placed in one long strip center with a vast sea of parking lots.

management The person or people who perform the act(s) of management: getting people to work together to accomplish desired goals and objectives efficiently and effectively.

manicurist The study and application of beauty treatment. Branches of specialty include treatment for the hands and feet.

medical spa A spa that is a cross between a medical clinic and a day spa, operating under the supervision of a medical doctor.

merchandising The methods, practices, and operations used to promote and sustain certain products and/or services within the business.

MSDS Material Safety Data Sheets.

multimedia Media and content that use a combination of different content forms, such as a combination of text, audio, still images, animation, video, and interactivity.

net profit The difference between the cost of goods and services and their selling price. Labor, as well as the shampoo and hair spray, would be part of the cost of a shampoo/style service.

NNN charges "Triple net" = Common area maintenance + Insurance for the shopping center + Real estate taxes for the shopping center.

nontipping A decision not to accept tips as a form of payment.

notary public A public officer constituted by law to serve the public in noncontentious matters usually concerned with estates, deeds, powers-of-attorney, and foreign and international business.

operating costs The day-to-day expenses incurred in running the business, such as sales and administration, as opposed to production.

overhead Also known as *operating expenses*; an ongoing expense of operating the business.

partnership A form of business in which two or more people operate for the common goal of making profit. Each partner has unlimited liability for all debts and profits of the business.

percentage clause A rent arrangement in which, after the salon and spa grosses a certain amount of business, the rent will be computed on a percentage of the gross sales.

permit A license granting certain rights, such as a construction permit, building permit, or repair permit, required in most areas for new or preexisting construction.

photocopy A photographic reproduction of any written, printed, or graphic material.

place of business A fixed establishment, temporary location, or place, including any mobile barber or beauty salon, in which one or more persons practice as barbers, hairstylists, cosmetologists, manicurists, or estheticians.

policies and procedures A set of documents that describe the business's policies for operation and the procedures designed to fulfill the policies.

power outage A short- or long-term loss of the electric power to an area. Also known as a *power cut, power failure, power loss,* or *blackout.*

privately owned salon and spa A business arrangement in which the owner has total and unlimited personal liability for profit or debts incurred by the business.

profit The positive financial gain, after all expenses have been subtracted, from an investment or business operation.

profit-sharing Various incentive plans that provide direct or indirect payments to employees that depend on the company's profitability, in addition to employees' regular salary and bonuses.

property tax A tax that a property owner is required to pay, determined by the value of the property owned.

public relations The maintenance and/or enhancement of a business's or organization's public image and reputation.

real profit The amount of money left after all bills have been paid.

receivables The amount due from individuals and companies. These are claims that are expected to be collected in cash.

reciprocity Interaction between two parties for mutual advantage .for example, A hairstylist maybe moving for one state to another and will require a new license. Some states will transfer those hours while others will require an additional hours or testing out before being issued a license in that state.

rent An agreed payment made periodically by a tenant to a landlord for the use of space, a building, a business, an office, and/or other property.

rental agreement A contractual arrangement between two parties where the landlord agrees to rent to the tenant for an agreed amount of time.

reoccurring debt Any debt or obligation that occurs on a continuing basis.

résumé A marketing tool used by individuals to secure a new job, most often containing a summary of relevant job experience and education.

retirement plan A special savings account, such as a 401(k) or Roth IRA, where an employee either defers part of his or her current income into a tax shelter, where it will grow tax-free until the employee withdraws it, or makes contributions into the account from after-tax income, where any gains on the principal are tax-free.

revenue Income that a company receives from the sale of goods and services to customers.

salary + commission A compensation arrangement in which, in addition to salary, a percentage of the money made from the provision of services is given back to the cosmetologist as income.

sales promotion Activities, materials, and techniques used to support the advertising and marketing/sales efforts of the business.

sales tax A consumption tax charged at the point of purchase for certain goods and services, usually calculated by applying a percentage rate to the taxable price of a sale.

S corporations For U.S. federal income-tax purposes, a corporation that makes a valid election to be taxed under Subchapter S of Chapter 1 of the Internal Revenue Code. In general, S corporations do not pay any federal income taxes. Instead, the corporation's income or losses are divided among and passed through to its shareholders.

search engines Web sites that search for information on the World Wide Web. The searches are presented in a list form and the results are often called "hits."

search-engine optimization The process of improving the visibility of a Web site in search engines.

security interest An interest payment used to secure the payment of a debt or obligation usually created by an agreement or in accordance to law.

sliding percentage Increasing or decreasing of a percentage of pay in accordance with a standard or a set of conditions normally designed to encourage staff productivity.

slogan A memorable motto or phrase used as a repetitive expression of an idea or purpose for the business.

social networking site An online platform or site that focuses on building and reflecting social relations among people who share interests and/or activities.

software The collection of computer programs and related data. This term was originally coined to contrast with the term *hardware* (meaning physical devices).

sole proprietorship A business arrangement in which a single individual owns all the assets of the business, including the profits generated by it, and assumes all responsibilities for any of the liabilities or debts.

sponsored ads An advertising product in which an ad appears next to the search results when people search for specific keywords.

sublicense A license giving rights to occupy a rented space to a person or company that is not the primary holder of such location.

tax The imposition of a financial charge or other levy upon a taxpayer (an individual or legal entity) by a state or the functional equivalent of a state such that failure to pay is punishable by law.

technician Someone who is in a technological field who has a understanding of the general theoretical principles of that field, such as a cosmetologist, manicurist, esthetician, or massage therapist.

temporary location A location that is not permanent for your business. A term that denotes a finite period of time, with a defined beginning and an end.

tentative contract A contract stating that, if the space can pass zoning rules and state board of cosmetology rules and regulations, and the salon and spa can get a permit for building and redecorating, an electrical permit, a plumbing permit, a sign permit, and any other permits that may be needed in that locality, on a given date, the owner of the salon and spa will sign the lease agreement.

tip report form A form that can be obtained by writing the local Internal Revenue Service (IRS) office. These forms are given to all employees, who are required to declare the amount of tips over a specified figure and return the form to the salon and spa owner/manager.

tip A compensation arrangement in which the client, to ensure prompt/proper service, gives a certain amount over and above the stated price of a service to the technician who performed the service. Cosmetologists often make a considerable portion of their income from client tips.

unsecured loans Commonly called *signature loans* or *personal loans*. Often, these types of loans are used for smaller purchases such as office equipment/computers.

use tax An excise tax levied by the government on otherwise "tax-free" goods purchased by a state resident for use, storage, or consumption within that resident's state. This tax does not apply to items for resale, and is used primarily for purchases made over the Internet and on out-of-state purchases where no sales tax is applied.

ventilation system The process of "changing" or replacing air in any space, often used as a device to control the temperature or remove moisture, odors, smoke, heat, dust, and so forth. Ventilation includes both the exchange of air to the outside as well as circulation of air within the business.

wages of nonproductive laborers Wages paid to employees who do not directly produce income—administrative staff, front desk associates, salon and spa managers, shampoo assistants, cleaning personnel (those who do not work on customers themselves), and repairmen (those who keep the equipment in working order).

wages of technicians Wages paid to productive workers who turn out a finished product—hairstylists, manicurists, estheticians, nail-care specialists, and massage therapists.

Web hosting A hosting service that allows the salon and spa site to be accessible via the World Wide Web.

Web site Web pages, images, and other information relative to a particular IP address. Primarily consisting solely of a domain name, it typically offers information about a subject, business, or service.

wet station Stations that are basically "all-in-one," designed to perform both wet and dry services.

word of mouth The passing of information from person to person. What once was literally words from the mouth now includes any type of social communication, such as Facebook, e-mail, text messaging, and telephone.

workers' compensation A form of insurance that provides compensation and medical care for employees who are injured in the course of employment, in exchange for mandatory relinquishment of the employee's right to sue his or her employer for the tort of negligence.

working capital Current assets minus current liabilities, measuring how much in liquid assets the business currently has available to build the business. This number will be affected positively or negatively by how much debt the company is currently carrying.

zip file A compressed file that takes up less storage space and therefore can be transferred to other computers quickly.

Salon and Spa Industry References

Web Sites

www.adweek.com

www.americanspa.com

www.beautyindustryprofessionals.com

www.beautyschoolsdirectory.com

www.cosmeticindustry.com

www.dayspamagazine.com/

www.dermascope.com

www.experienceispa.com

www.gcimagazine.com/

www.healthy-holistic-living.com

www.lohas.com

www.spahub.com/

www.magazine.com

www.marketingpower.com/

www.massageandbodywork.com

www.nouvelles-esthetiques.com

www.salontoday.com

www.skininc.com

www.spabeautyschool.com

www.spafinder.com

www.spamagazine.com

www.spamanagement.com

www.womanowned.com

www.yellowpages.com

Journals

American Demographics

Beauty School Directory

Cosmetic Surgery Times

DAYSPA

Global Cosmetic Industry

LOHAS

Luxury Spa Finder

Marketing News (AMA)

Massage & Body work

Medical Spa Report

nouvelles-esthetiques.com

Pulse (ISPA)

Salon Today

Skin, Inc.

Spa Finder

Spa Healthy Living Travel & Renewal

Spa Management

spabeautyschool.com

spafinder.com

Women's Business

Organizations

American Advertising Federation

American Association of Advertising Agencies

American Business Brokers Association

American Institute of Architects (AIA)

American Institute of Certified Public Accountants

American Marketing Association

American Society of Aesthetic Plastic Surgery

American Society of Appraisers

Better Business Bureau

Day Spa Association (DSA)

Federation of Tax Administrators

Green Spa Network

International Spa Association (ISPA)

National Association of Certified Valuation Analysis

National Association of Woman Business Owners (NAWBO)

National Coalition of Estheticians, Manufactures/ Distributors & Associations (NCEA)

Small Business Service Bureau

Spa Association (SPAA)

U.S. Government Agencies

Bureau of Economic Census

Bureau of Labor Statistics

Census Bureau

Centers for Disease Control (CDC)

Consumer Product Safety Commission (CPSC)

Department of Commerce (DOC)

Department of Education (DOE)

Department of Health and Human Services (HHS)

Department of Justice (DOJ)

Department of Labor (DOL)

Department of Revenue (DOR)

Department of Treasury, Internal Revenue Service (IRS)

Environmental Protection Agency (EPA)

Equal Opportunity Employment Commission (EEOC)

Federal Trade Commission (FTC)

Food and Drug Administration (FDA)

Immigration and Naturalization Services (INS)

Internal Revenue Service (IRS)

National Center for Complementary and Alternative Medicine (NCAM)

National Trademark Office (U.S. Patent and Trademark Office)

Occupational Safety and Health Administration (OSHA)

Small Business Administration (SBA)

Index